Force Your Fat to Melt: A Transformation Guide to Nutrition

Abstract

"The Nutrition and Fat Burning Guide" offers a comprehensive resource for individuals looking to adopt a healthy lifestyle and optimize fat burning. The book thoroughly examines the effects of nutrition, exercise, and lifestyle factors on fat loss while providing readers with information grounded in scientific principles.

Focusing on the importance of fat burning for health, the book debunks common myths and reveals the truth. It delves into topics such as metabolism, calorie balance, and the role of macronutrients, ensuring readers have access to accurate information. Additionally, practical insights are provided on setting healthy body composition goals, understanding protein requirements, and recognizing the significance of healthy fats.

The guide also addresses the flexibility and sustainability of nutrition programs, modern dietary approaches like intermittent fasting, and the impact of whole foods and supplements on fat burning. It highlights how exercise programs can support fat loss, the benefits of HIIT workouts, and methods for increasing daily mobility.

Finally, topics such as adopting healthy habits, making healthy choices in social settings, and maintaining long-term motivation are discussed to help readers develop the strategies they will need on their journey to a healthier life.

This guide aims not only to help readers achieve their weight loss goals but also to encourage the adoption of a lasting and healthy lifestyle. Healthy living should be embraced as a way of life, not just a goal. "The Nutrition and Fat Burning Guide" serves as a resource to guide readers on this journey.

Introduction

In today's world, healthy living has become not just a goal but also a lifestyle. Rapidly changing living conditions significantly affect our eating habits and overall health. Many of us may struggle with maintaining healthy nutrition and adequate physical activity amidst busy work lives, stressful days, and a fast-paced lifestyle. However, it should be noted that living a healthy life is not limited to physical appearance; it also encompasses mental and emotional well-being.

The purpose of this book is to help you understand the fundamental principles of nutrition and fat burning. While exploring the requirements of healthy living, we want to emphasize not only the importance of achieving your weight loss goals but also adopting a healthy lifestyle.

Understanding the balance between nutrition, exercise, and lifestyle factors is critical to improving your individual health.

Fat burning is not just an aesthetic goal but a vital process for our health. Keeping body fat levels in check contributes to proper metabolic function, maintaining heart health, and enhancing overall quality of life. In this book, we will deeply explore why fat burning is so important for healthy living, helping you access accurate information by debunking common myths.

This book serves as a guide enriched with current scientific research and practical information. By covering topics such as macronutrients, micronutrients, calorie balance, types of exercise, and mental health, we aim to provide all the knowledge needed to lead a healthy life. We will also explore ways to develop healthy habits and examine issues of flexibility and sustainability.

As you embark on this journey, remember to be gentle with yourself and stay open to learning at every step. Healthy living is not a destination but a continuous journey. This book will guide you along that journey and help you embrace a healthy lifestyle. Now, are you ready to take the first steps on your healthy living journey?

1. Healthy Living and Fat Burning

The Importance of Fat Burning for Healthy Living

Fat burning is not merely an aesthetic goal; it is vital for the maintenance and improvement of overall health. Excess fat accumulation in the body, particularly visceral fat surrounding internal organs, can increase the risk of chronic diseases. A lifestyle that promotes fat burning helps improve cardiovascular health, maintain metabolic balance, and elevate overall energy levels.

Protection Against Chronic Diseases

Obesity is directly associated with various chronic conditions, including type 2 diabetes, hypertension, cardiovascular diseases, and certain types of cancer (World Health Organization [WHO], 2020). Research shows that reducing body fat percentage is effective in lowering the risks associated with these diseases (Nguyen & El-Serag, 2010). In particular, the reduction of visceral fat allows organs to function more healthily, which opens the doors to a healthier life in the long run.

Improving Metabolic Health

Controlling body fat percentage can enhance insulin sensitivity and prevent disorders such as metabolic syndrome. During fat burning, the body meets its energy needs from fat tissues, which helps stabilize blood sugar and insulin levels. This process leads to a more balanced energy metabolism, reduces fatigue, and promotes a greater sense of vitality throughout the day (Saltiel & Olefsky, 2017).

Effects on Physical Performance and Fitness

Reducing body fat to achieve a leaner physique makes daily physical activities easier. Fat burning helps preserve muscle mass and supports muscle development while also contributing to endurance and strength gains (McArdle, Katch, & Katch, 2010). Fat loss, supported by regular exercise, enhances bodily flexibility, movement capacity, and overall physical performance.

Psychological Health and Self-Confidence

The vitality gained through fat loss can have positive effects on psychological health. Neurotransmitters released during exercise, such as endorphins, can help reduce symptoms of depression and anxiety (Craft & Perna, 2004). Additionally, achieving targeted fat loss increases feelings of personal accomplishment and boosts self-confidence. Having a healthy body composition can help individuals feel better in their social and professional lives and achieve higher levels of motivation.

Fat burning is not solely about weight loss; it is also a critical element for overall health, metabolic balance, and mental well-being. In this regard, adopting a sustainable lifestyle can contribute to individuals leading healthier lives and enhancing their quality of life.

Common Myths and Facts About Fat Burning

Fat burning is a popular goal for many people seeking a healthy body composition and balanced weight. However, many misconceptions lacking scientific basis have proliferated in this area. These myths can hinder healthy weight management and even harm health. Here are some of the most common myths and scientific facts about fat burning:

1. **Myth:** "Only Cardio Exercises Are Necessary for Fat Burning."
   Fact: While cardio exercises contribute to fat burning, resistance training aimed at increasing muscle mass is also critical for fat loss. Resistance training increases muscle mass, which raises basal metabolic rate, leading to more calories burned even at rest (Westcott, 2012). A balanced combination of cardio and resistance exercises is more effective for long-term fat loss.
2. **Myth:** "You Can Burn Fat by Starving Yourself."
   Fact: While it may be possible to lose weight in the short term by starving yourself or following very low-calorie diets, this approach is unhealthy. Low-calorie diets can lead to muscle loss and decreased metabolic rate, making long-term weight management more challenging (Dulloo et al., 1997). Consuming a balanced diet with adequate protein, carbohydrates, and healthy fats is more effective for sustainable fat loss.

3. **Myth:** "You Need to Eat Fat-Free to Burn Fat."
   Fact: Eating a fat-free diet can disrupt the body's energy balance and hormone levels. Healthy fats support cell membrane structure, hormone production, and the absorption of fat-soluble vitamins (Willett, 2012). Healthy fat sources, such as avocados, nuts, and olive oil, can support weight loss and fat burning when consumed in controlled portions.

4. **Myth:** "Fat Burning Can Be Targeted to Specific Areas" (Spot Reduction).
   Fact: The body loses fat evenly from all areas, and spot reduction is not possible. For example, performing sit-ups to lose fat from the abdominal area does not accelerate fat burning in that region. Fat loss can occur at different rates in various areas of the body, depending on factors such as genetics, age, and gender (Vispute et al., 2011). However, regular exercise and a healthy diet can help reduce overall body fat.

5. **Myth:** "Metabolic Rate Is Fixed and Cannot Be Changed."
   Fact: Metabolic rate is influenced by age, gender, and genetic factors, but it can also be increased through lifestyle changes. Resistance exercises and regular physical activity can be effective in boosting metabolic rate. Additionally, the thermic effect of protein consumption is high, meaning that more energy is expended for protein digestion (Hume et al., 2016). Therefore, a balanced diet and an active lifestyle can positively impact metabolic rate.

6. **Myth:** "Eating at Night Causes Weight Gain."
   Fact: There is no scientific evidence that eating at night directly leads to weight gain; what matters is total daily calorie intake and energy balance. However, consuming heavy, fatty, or sugary foods late at night can disrupt sleep patterns and complicate digestion. Research suggests that calorie control and balanced nutrition are more effective for weight management than meal timing (Swinburn et al., 2011).

7. **Myth:** "Just Dieting Is Enough for Fat Burning."
   Fact: Diet alone is not sufficient for achieving a healthy body composition; it should be supported by regular exercise. While diet helps control calorie intake to support fat loss, exercise promotes the preservation of muscle mass and speeds up metabolism (Jakicic et al., 2001). The most effective fat burning occurs with regular physical activity alongside a balanced diet.

8. **Myth:** "Detox Diets Accelerate Fat Burning."
   Fact: There is no scientific evidence that detox diets directly burn body fat. While these diets often lead to short-term weight loss due to being low in calories, they do not create lasting effects in the long term. Additionally, the body has a natural detoxification process through organs like the liver and kidneys (Klein & Kiat, 2015). A balanced and nutritious diet should be preferred for sustainable weight loss.

Having accurate information about fat burning is essential for sustainable and healthy weight management. Moving beyond myths and opting for scientifically supported methods helps protect both physical and mental health. For a healthy life, the importance of balanced nutrition and regular physical activity is significant.

The Impact of Nutrition, Exercise, and Lifestyle Factors on Fat Burning

Fat burning occurs through the combination of various factors to achieve energy balance and a healthy body composition. Among the most significant elements affecting this process are nutrition, regular exercise, and healthy lifestyle habits. Each of these factors has different impacts on the body's fat storage and burning mechanisms.

1. **The Role of Nutrition in Fat Burning**
   Nutrition plays a critical role in fat burning because the amount of calories consumed and the distribution of nutrients directly affect the body's energy balance.
   - **Caloric Balance**: Creating a caloric deficit is essential for fat burning; in other words, one must consume fewer calories than the body needs. However, an excessive deficit can lead to muscle loss and a decrease in metabolic rate, so a balanced caloric deficit should be targeted (Hall et al., 2011).
   - **Macronutrient Distribution**: Consuming adequate amounts of protein is important for preserving muscle mass and boosting metabolism. High protein intake supports fat burning through its thermic effect (the energy expended during digestion) (Leidy et al., 2015). A balanced ratio of carbohydrates and healthy fats also helps maintain energy levels.
   - **Fiber and Water Intake**: Foods rich in fiber can increase feelings of fullness, preventing unnecessary calorie intake. Additionally, water consumption supports the body's metabolic processes and contributes to fat burning (Stookey et al., 2008).

2. **The Impact of Exercise on Fat Burning**
   Regular physical activity accelerates fat loss and improves body composition while preserving muscle mass.
   - **Cardio Exercises**: High-Intensity Interval Training (HIIT) provides high calorie burn in a shorter time compared to traditional cardio exercises. Furthermore, it has been shown that fat burning continues for some time after HIIT (Boutcher, 2011).
   - **Resistance Training**: Resistance exercises like weight lifting help increase muscle mass, leading to higher calorie burn even at rest, contributing to fat loss in the long term (Schoenfeld, 2010).
   - **Daily Activity**: Besides exercising, staying active throughout the day is important. Increasing daily movement (such as taking short walks or using the stairs) supports fat burning and boosts metabolism (Levine, 2002).

3. **The Impact of Lifestyle Factors on Fat Burning**
   In addition to nutrition and exercise, lifestyle factors significantly affect fat burning. Sleep patterns, stress management, and overall lifestyle habits play a crucial role in the body's fat burning capacity.
   - **Sleep Patterns**: Adequate and quality sleep helps maintain metabolism and ensures the healthy functioning of appetite-regulating hormones (leptin and

ghrelin). Studies show that sleep deprivation can lead to weight gain and hinder fat loss (Chaput et al., 2007).

- ○ **Stress Management**: Chronic stress can lead to increased cortisol levels, resulting in greater fat storage. Keeping cortisol levels in check, especially to avoid abdominal fat accumulation, supports fat loss. Stress-reducing activities like meditation, deep breathing exercises, or hobbies can aid this process (Epel et al., 2001).
- ○ **Alcohol Consumption**: Alcohol is a high-calorie beverage and can slow down the body's fat-burning process. Regular and excessive alcohol consumption, particularly, disrupts the liver's fat-burning function and increases fat storage. Therefore, limiting alcohol intake is important for fat loss goals (Suter et al., 1997).

To support fat burning, it is essential to address nutrition, exercise, and lifestyle factors together. A healthy eating plan, regular physical activity, and balanced lifestyle habits allow the body to sustainably increase fat loss. This holistic approach not only supports weight loss but also improves the individual's overall health and quality of life.

What Readers Will Gain from the Book and Motivation Provision
This book aims to help readers not only lose weight but also make profound and healthy changes in their lifestyles. The information, recommendations, and tips provided throughout the book will equip readers with in-depth knowledge about healthy eating, exercise, and lifestyle habits, enabling them to integrate this information into their daily lives.

What Readers Will Gain

- **Knowledge and Awareness**: Readers will gain scientific knowledge about fat burning, healthy weight management, and nutrition. By learning about common myths and facts, they will develop a correct perspective, which will help them set long-term, sustainable health goals.
- **Self-Confidence and Control**: Every step taken toward a healthy lifestyle contributes to the individual's understanding of their body, knowledge of their limits, and increased self-confidence. The book will provide tools to develop willpower and support readers in achieving their goals, reinforcing a sense of personal control.
- **Practical Application in Daily Life**: Theoretical information will be supported by practical recommendations, detailing how readers can apply what they learn to their daily lives step by step. This approach will facilitate making the acquired knowledge a part of life, enabling a sustainable healthy lifestyle.
- **Mental and Physical Health**: The book will emphasize not only physical changes but also mental health. Healthy eating and exercise habits have positive effects on mood and overall happiness. Readers will strengthen mentally as well as physically.

- **Higher Energy Levels**: Healthy eating and regular physical activity enhance energy levels, allowing individuals to feel more efficient and energetic in their daily lives. Readers will see an increase in their physical and mental performance with these new habits they incorporate into their lives.

Motivation Provision

Throughout the book, various strategies will be employed to enhance motivation and inspire readers:

- **Real-Life Examples and Success Stories**: The book will feature stories of individuals who have achieved success on their healthy living journeys. These stories will boost readers' confidence and motivate them.
- **Motivational Quotes and Sayings**: Each chapter will share inspiring quotes and motivational sayings to support readers in their healthy living journey. This will help readers find small support in every page of the book.
- **Setting Small Goals and Celebrating Success**: Readers will be informed about the importance of setting small, achievable goals on the path to larger objectives. They will be encouraged to reward themselves at every step of success, helping maintain motivation.
- **Positive Language and Affirmative Guidance**: The tone of the book will be supportive, encouraging, and action-oriented. Techniques for overcoming challenges and motivation for overcoming obstacles will also be shared.

With the information and strategies presented in this book, readers will learn not only to lose weight but also to make a sustainable healthy lifestyle. By staying motivated and progressing steadily on their healthy living journeys, they will achieve long-term success.

2. Understanding Fat Burning

What is Metabolism and Metabolic Rate, and How is it Affected?

Metabolism refers to all the chemical processes that the body undergoes to survive and maintain its functions. These processes allow the body to produce energy, renew cells, and carry out all biological functions necessary for life. Understanding the various factors that influence metabolism is essential for fat burning and weight management.

What is Metabolism and Metabolic Rate?

Metabolism: This is the process by which the body breaks down food to convert it into energy, enabling it to function. This energy facilitates the occurrence of chemical reactions between cells, maintains body temperature, regulates heartbeats, supports breathing, and fulfills other vital functions. In short, metabolism is a system in which the body is in a constant cycle of energy production to survive.

Metabolic Rate: Metabolic rate refers to the number of calories the body burns while at rest. In other words, it indicates the amount of energy required for the body to maintain its basic functions. When measured at rest, this rate is called the basal metabolic rate (BMR) and varies from individual to individual. Metabolic rate is an important determinant for weight management and fat burning, as it indicates the amount of energy the body needs (Müller et al., 2011).

Factors Affecting Metabolic Rate

Many different factors influence metabolic rate, ranging from a person's genetic makeup to their age, dietary habits, and level of physical activity. Here are some key factors that affect metabolic rate:

- **Genetic Factors:** A person's genetic makeup has a significant impact on metabolic rate. Some individuals naturally have a faster metabolism, while others have a slower metabolism. Genetics determine a portion of metabolic rate but are not entirely modifiable (Bouchard et al., 1990).
- **Age:** Metabolism tends to slow down as a person ages. Typically, after the age of 30, metabolic rate decreases due to a reduction in muscle mass and hormonal changes. This can lead to a tendency to gain weight as one ages (Gurven & Kaplan, 2007).
- **Gender:** Women's body composition typically differs from men's, with women generally having a higher percentage of body fat. Men usually have more muscle mass, which raises their metabolic rates. As muscle mass increases, so does metabolic rate (De Lorenzo et al., 1999).
- **Muscle Mass:** The more muscle mass a person has, the higher their metabolic rate. Muscle tissue burns more energy compared to fat tissue. Therefore, individuals with a higher muscle ratio tend to have higher metabolic rates (Speakman & Selman, 2003).
- **Dietary Habits:** Eating habits can also influence metabolic rate. Low-calorie diets or prolonged periods of fasting can slow down metabolism, as the body shifts into a conservation mode during hunger. Regular, balanced meals support metabolic function (Müller et al., 2011).
- **Physical Activity:** Engaging in regular exercise is one of the most effective ways to boost metabolism. High-Intensity Interval Training (HIIT) and resistance training, in particular, revitalize metabolism both during and after exercise. They also help preserve metabolic rate over the long term by increasing muscle mass (Heden et al., 2015).
- **Hormones:** Hormones such as thyroid hormones directly affect metabolism. For example, a reduction in thyroid hormones can slow down metabolic rate. Similarly, insulin, cortisol, and growth hormones can also influence metabolism (Blum et al., 2011).

- **Sleep Patterns and Stress:** Lack of sleep and chronic stress can negatively affect metabolic rate. The body rests during sleep, and hormone levels stabilize. Insufficient sleep can influence hunger hormones, increasing appetite and potentially leading to weight gain (Knutson et al., 2007). Under stress, the body tends to store fat by increasing cortisol hormone levels (Epel et al., 2001).

Recommendations for Increasing Metabolic Rate

To naturally increase metabolic rate and support fat burning, consider the following recommendations:

- **Exercise Regularly:** Especially focus on exercises that build muscle mass and HIIT, as they contribute to an increase in metabolic rate.
- **Eat a Balanced Diet and Don't Skip Meals:** Maintain energy balance with regular meals and avoid going hungry. Skipping meals can slow down metabolism.
- **Consume Enough Protein:** Protein is a nutrient with a high thermic effect and requires more energy to digest.
- **Drink Plenty of Water:** Water supports metabolic activities and contributes to energy production.
- **Maintain a Sleep Routine:** Getting adequate and quality sleep each night ensures that metabolism functions healthily.

Understanding and supporting metabolic rate is crucial for healthy weight management and fat burning. Making lifestyle changes that consider these factors creates a strong foundation for achieving long-term health goals.

Difference Between Weight Loss and Fat Burning

Weight loss and fat burning are terms often used interchangeably; however, there are significant differences between these concepts. While both are considered parts of a healthy lifestyle, they differ in terms of goals, processes, and outcomes.

Weight Loss

Weight loss refers to a decrease in an individual's total body weight. This can involve loss of different components in the body, such as fat, water, and muscle tissue. The following elements are considered in the weight loss process:

- **Weight Components:** Weight loss includes not only fat loss but also the loss of water and muscle mass. Rapid weight loss often starts with water loss, which can have adverse health effects.
- **Short-Term Goals:** Weight loss typically focuses on short-term goals. It may be pursued to change appearance quickly for a specific event or date.

- **Diet and Exercise Programs:** Weight loss is usually achieved through calorie-restrictive diets and increased physical activity. However, the emphasis is on total weight loss rather than fat loss.
- **Quick Results:** Some diet programs promise rapid weight loss within a short period. However, these methods are often unsustainable, and lost weight can be regained (Vickers et al., 2016).

Fat Burning

Fat burning refers to the reduction of fat tissue in the body. This process involves the body using stored fats to meet its energy needs. Key points about fat burning include:

- **Fat Components:** Fat burning involves the utilization of stored fats in the body. Fat loss forms the basis of a healthy weight loss process and is generally a more sustainable goal.
- **Long-Term Goals:** Fat burning typically focuses on long-term goals. The aim is to improve body composition, reduce body fat percentage, and preserve muscle mass.
- **Nutrition and Exercise Strategies:** Fat burning is supported by a balanced diet and a regular exercise program. Specifically, strength training and aerobic activities are effective in increasing fat burning (Stannard & Johnstone, 2004).
- **Sustainable Results:** The fat burning process generally leads to more sustainable outcomes. Slow and steady fat loss improves the body's health while supporting the individual's metabolism.

While weight loss and fat burning share similar goals, they offer different approaches and outcomes. Weight loss is defined as a reduction in total weight, while fat burning refers to using fats as energy to improve body composition and maintain a healthy lifestyle. The goal for a healthy life is not only to lose weight but also to promote fat burning and preserve muscle mass. Therefore, it is important to adopt a sustainable approach that includes healthy eating and regular physical activity when pursuing weight loss goals.

Setting Healthy Body Composition Goals

A healthy body composition refers to a balanced distribution of fat, muscle, water, and other components in the body. Setting body composition goals is a critical step toward achieving personal health, fitness, and aesthetic aspirations. Here are key elements to consider when setting healthy body composition goals:

1. **Define Your Goals**
   - **Weight Goals:** Determine your goals regarding weight loss, weight gain, or maintaining your current weight. While setting your goals, ensure you remain within a healthy weight range.

- ○ **Body Fat Percentage:** Reducing or increasing body fat percentage may be part of your healthy body composition goals. A body fat percentage of 10-20% for men and 20-30% for women is generally considered healthy (Nindl et al., 2007).
  - ○ **Muscle Mass:** Increasing muscle mass supports fat burning by speeding up metabolism. Focusing on muscle development provides a firmer and fitter appearance.

2. **Set Realistic and Measurable Goals**
   - ○ **SMART Goals:** When determining your goals, ensure they align with SMART criteria (Specific, Measurable, Achievable, Realistic, Time-bound). For instance, you could set a specific and measurable goal like, "I aim to lose 3 kilograms of fat in three months."

3. **Assess Body Composition**
   - ○ **Body Mass Index (BMI):** BMI indicates how healthy your weight is relative to your height. However, it is not sufficient to rely solely on BMI; evaluating other aspects of body composition is also important.
   - ○ **Body Fat Measurements:** There are various methods to determine body fat percentage. Techniques such as bioelectrical impedance analysis (BIA), skinfold thickness measurement, or DEXA scans can assess body fat percentage (Heymsfield et al., 1990).

4. **Create Nutrition and Exercise Plans**
   - ○ **Balanced Nutrition:** It is crucial to develop a balanced nutrition plan for a healthy body composition. Consider the balance of carbohydrates, proteins, and fats. Consuming sufficient protein helps maintain and increase muscle mass.
   - ○ **Physical Activity:** Establish a fitness program that includes aerobic and resistance exercises. At least 150 minutes of moderate-intensity aerobic activity and muscle-strengthening exercises on two days per week are recommended (WHO, 2020).

5. **Monitor and Evaluate Progress**
   - ○ **Regular Check-Ups:** Regularly review your body composition and goals. Assess your progress monthly or quarterly. Seeing whether you are making strides toward your goals can enhance your motivation.
   - ○ **Make Adjustments:** If you find it challenging to reach your goals, review your nutrition or exercise program. Seek support from a nutritionist or fitness expert to guide your changes effectively.

Setting healthy body composition goals involves more than just focusing on weight. A comprehensive plan that considers body fat percentage, muscle mass, and overall health will lead to a healthier lifestyle. It is important to adopt realistic and achievable goals, monitor progress, and adjust strategies as necessary to maintain a balanced approach to body composition.

3. Principles of Proper Nutrition for Fat Burning

Information on Caloric Balance and Energy Intake

Caloric balance and energy intake are fundamental elements that affect body weight, body composition, and overall health. These concepts are critical for maintaining a healthy lifestyle and managing weight.

What is Caloric Balance?

Caloric balance refers to the equilibrium between the number of calories consumed and the number of calories expended. There are three primary states of caloric balance:

- **Energy Balance:** Achieved when the number of calories consumed equals the number of calories expended. In this case, body weight remains stable.
- **Energy Surplus:** Occurs when calorie intake exceeds calorie expenditure. This leads to weight gain, as excess calories are stored as fat in the body.
- **Energy Deficit:** Happens when calorie intake is less than calorie expenditure. This results in weight loss, as the body starts using stored fat and muscle for energy needs.

Energy Intake

Energy intake refers to the number of calories obtained from the food and beverages consumed to meet daily energy needs. Energy intake is influenced by several factors:

- **Individual Differences:** Each person's caloric needs vary based on age, gender, weight, height, and level of physical activity. For instance, an active individual requires more calories than a sedentary one (Müller et al., 2014).
- **Basal Metabolic Rate (BMR):** The energy expended by the body at rest (such as during sleep). BMR is the minimum amount of energy required to sustain vital bodily functions. It is influenced by factors like genetics, age, gender, and muscle mass (Rogers et al., 2016).
- **Physical Activity:** Daily physical activities, sports, and exercise increase total energy expenditure. Regular exercise also boosts BMR by increasing muscle mass.
- **Thermic Effect:** The amount of energy expended during the digestion, absorption, and metabolism of food. The digestion of proteins requires more energy compared to fats and carbohydrates. Therefore, a protein-rich diet contributes to higher calorie burn through the thermic effect (Westerterp, 2004).

Managing Caloric Intake

Managing caloric intake is essential for maintaining a healthy lifestyle and achieving ideal body weight. Here are some key considerations:

- **Balanced Nutrition:** Create a meal plan that considers the balance of carbohydrates, proteins, and fats. Focus on natural and nutrient-rich foods while avoiding processed foods.
- **Portion Control:** Monitoring portion sizes can help prevent excessive calorie intake. Using smaller plates and eating slowly and mindfully can aid in this effort.
- **Increase Physical Activity:** Regular exercise can help you achieve a healthy caloric balance by increasing calorie expenditure. Don't forget to incorporate strength training activities along with aerobic exercises.
- **Monitoring and Evaluation:** Keeping track of your daily caloric intake can help you reach your goals. Maintaining a food diary or using mobile apps allows you to evaluate your caloric intake and expenditure.

Caloric balance and energy intake are vital for maintaining a healthy lifestyle and managing weight. Balanced nutrition, regular physical activity, and monitoring caloric intake are important steps for individuals to achieve their health goals. Adopting a healthy lifestyle is essential not only for weight management but also for overall health and well-being.

Macronutrients: Carbohydrates, Proteins, Fats

Macronutrients encompass the three main food groups essential for meeting the body's energy needs and maintaining healthy functioning: carbohydrates, proteins, and fats. Each macronutrient plays unique roles in various bodily functions, and consuming them in appropriate balances is crucial for health.

1. **Carbohydrates**

   Carbohydrates are one of the most important energy sources for the body and are generally recommended to make up 45-65% of daily caloric intake (Institute of Medicine, 2005).
   - **Types:**
     - **Simple Carbohydrates:** Known as sugars, these consist of single or double sugar units, such as glucose and fructose. They provide quick energy but can lead to rapid fluctuations in blood sugar levels. Examples include honey, sugar, and fruits.
     - **Complex Carbohydrates:** These structures contain multiple sugar units and are found in forms such as starch and fiber. They provide longer-lasting energy due to their slower digestion. Examples include whole grains, legumes, and vegetables.
   - **Benefits:**

- Provide a quick source of energy.
- Fiber-rich carbohydrates support digestion and improve gut health.

2. Proteins

Proteins are the building blocks of the body and play a critical role in the formation of muscles, skin, hair, and enzymes. It is recommended that 10-35% of daily caloric intake comes from proteins (Institute of Medicine, 2005).

- **Types:**
  - **Complete Proteins:** These proteins contain all essential amino acids and typically come from animal sources. Examples include meat, dairy products, and eggs.
  - **Complementary Proteins:** These plant-based protein sources do not contain all essential amino acids but can complement each other when consumed together. An example is the combination of grains and legumes (e.g., rice and beans).
- **Benefits:**
  - Necessary for maintaining and developing muscle mass.
  - Assists in body repair and growth.
  - Plays an important role in hormonal and enzymatic functions.

3. Fats

Fats are the body's form of energy storage and are recommended to constitute 20-35% of daily caloric intake (Institute of Medicine, 2005). Fats not only provide energy but also contribute to cell structure and hormone production.

- **Types:**
  - **Saturated Fats:** Typically derived from animal sources, these fats are usually solid at room temperature. Excessive consumption can negatively affect heart health. Examples include butter and full-fat dairy products.
  - **Unsaturated Fats:** Considered healthy fats, these come from sources like olive oil, avocado, and nuts. They have supportive effects on heart health.
    - **Monounsaturated Fats:** Come from sources such as olive oil and avocados.
    - **Polyunsaturated Fats:** Include healthy fats like omega-3 and omega-6 fatty acids found in foods such as fish, walnuts, and chia seeds.
  - **Trans Fats:** Found mainly in processed foods, these fats are harmful to health and should be avoided. Examples include margarine and some fast food items.
- **Benefits:**
  - Provide energy and assist in the absorption of fat-soluble vitamins (A, D, E, K).
  - Support hormonal balance and brain health.

Carbohydrates, proteins, and fats are the fundamental elements of a healthy nutrition plan. Each macronutrient assumes different roles for bodily functionality and health. A balanced diet requires the appropriate consumption of these three macronutrients. By developing healthy eating habits, it is possible to make the most of these macronutrients. It is important to remember that each individual's nutritional needs are different, and it is best to create a diet plan tailored to personal goals.

The Importance of Micronutrients: Vitamins, Minerals, Antioxidants

Micronutrients are nutrients such as vitamins, minerals, and antioxidants that are essential for the healthy functioning of the body but need to be consumed in only small amounts. These micronutrients support the body's metabolism, strengthen the immune system, and provide protection against various diseases. Below, the main components of micronutrients and their effects on health are detailed.

1. **Vitamins** Vitamins are organic compounds that support various functions in the body and are generally divided into two groups:
    - **Fat-Soluble Vitamins:** Vitamins A, D, E, and K can be found in fatty foods because they are soluble in fat and can be stored in the body. These vitamins play crucial roles in enhancing the immune system, supporting cell health, and contributing to bone health.
    - **Water-Soluble Vitamins:** Vitamins that dissolve in water, such as vitamin C and the B vitamins, cannot be stored in the body and must be consumed regularly. These vitamins are essential for energy production, nervous system health, and immune function (Hoffman et al., 2013).

Benefits:

- Vitamins play a significant role in metabolic processes and act as coenzymes for many biochemical reactions.
- They enhance the immune system, increasing resistance to diseases.
- They improve skin and eye health and elevate energy levels.
2. **Minerals** Minerals are inorganic compounds that serve many important functions in the body. The essential minerals required by the body include:
    - **Macrominerals:** Minerals such as calcium, phosphorus, potassium, magnesium, sodium, and chloride are found in large amounts in the body and have significant functions. For example, calcium is critical for bone health (Weaver, 2013).
    - **Trace Elements:** Minerals like iron, zinc, copper, manganese, iodine, and selenium are present in smaller amounts but perform vital functions. For example, iron is necessary for hemoglobin, which carries oxygen.

Benefits:

- Minerals regulate cellular functions and contribute to enzyme activation.
- They help maintain electrolyte balance and fluid balance.
- They are essential for muscle function and nerve transmission.

3. **Antioxidants** Antioxidants are compounds that protect cells from oxidative stress by combating free radicals. Many vitamins and minerals found in nature exhibit antioxidant properties. Key antioxidants include:
    - **Vitamin C:** Soluble in water and plays many vital roles in the body, particularly for immune system and skin health.
    - **Vitamin E:** A fat-soluble vitamin that protects cell membranes and supports skin health.
    - **Selenium:** This trace element supports the function of antioxidant enzymes and helps strengthen the immune system (Rayman, 2012).

Benefits:

- Protects cell health by reducing the effects of oxidative stress.
- May lower the risk of chronic diseases, cancers, and age-related illnesses.
- Enhances the immune system, increasing resistance to diseases.

Micronutrients are vital for a healthy life. Vitamins, minerals, and antioxidants regulate the body's metabolism, support the immune system, and create positive effects on overall health. A balanced and varied diet is necessary to ensure adequate intake of these micronutrients. Foods rich in micronutrients, such as fruits, vegetables, whole grains, nuts, and legumes, form the foundation of a healthy diet. Therefore, developing healthy eating habits to increase micronutrient intake is a critical step for overall health and well-being.

Flexibility and Sustainability in Nutrition Programs

Nutrition programs help individuals adopt a healthy lifestyle, with flexibility and sustainability as key elements. A flexible and sustainable approach to nutrition provides positive effects on both physical and psychological health, facilitating individuals' long-term goals.

1. **Flexibility** Flexibility in nutrition programs allows individuals to be open to different food options and make healthy choices without strict dietary restrictions. Several key elements of a flexible nutrition approach include:
    - **Variety:** Including a variety of foods in the nutrition program is essential for obtaining all necessary nutrients. Vegetables and fruits of different colors, whole grains, and protein sources create a nutritionally rich diet (López-Olmeda et al., 2020).

- ○ **Emotional and Social Eating:** Meals are a part of social interactions and emotional experiences. A flexible nutrition approach allows individuals to enjoy delicious foods on special occasions or in social settings while helping them maintain their healthy habits (Davis et al., 2016).
  - ○ **Individual Preferences and Needs:** Each individual has different nutritional needs and preferences. A flexible approach enables individuals to develop a personalized nutrition program tailored to their needs, allowing them to stay healthy sustainably.

2. **Sustainability** A sustainable nutrition program helps meet individual health needs while minimizing environmental impacts. Components of a sustainable diet include:
   - ○ **Local and Seasonal Foods:** Consuming local and seasonal products reduces the environmental impact of the food system and enhances the freshness of food. Foods consumed in season are often more nutritious and flavorful (Smith et al., 2014).
   - ○ **Plant-Based Nutrition:** Making plant-based foods (vegetables, fruits, legumes, grains) the foundation of the diet is essential for environmental sustainability. Plant-based foods are associated with lower greenhouse gas emissions compared to animal-based foods and reduce ecological footprints (Willett et al., 2019).
   - ○ **Reducing Food Waste:** A sustainable nutrition program includes strategies to minimize food waste. By shopping with a plan and utilizing leftover food, both economic and environmental benefits can be achieved.

3. **Creating a Flexible and Sustainable Nutrition Program** To create a flexible and sustainable nutrition program, the following steps can be taken:
   - ○ **Goal Setting:** Identifying personal health goals is the first step in creating a sustainable diet. Goals such as weight loss, increasing energy, or improving overall health can guide appropriate food choices.
   - ○ **Planning and Preparation:** Creating weekly meal plans promotes the consumption of healthy and diverse foods. Preparing in advance makes it easier to find healthy alternatives to unhealthy snacks.
   - ○ **Mindful Eating:** Understanding how emotional and social factors affect eating supports a flexible nutrition approach. Individuals can better manage their eating habits and preferences.
   - ○ **Environmental Awareness:** Prioritizing local and sustainable food sources while considering the environmental impact of the nutrition program contributes not only to a healthy diet but also to the protection of the planet.

Flexibility and sustainability are fundamental components of nutrition programs. These elements facilitate individuals' adoption of healthy eating habits while also reducing environmental impacts. Establishing a healthy and balanced diet improves individuals' overall health and represents an important step towards environmental sustainability. Therefore, adopting flexible and sustainable approaches in nutrition programs helps maintain a healthy lifestyle sustainably.

4. Distribution of Macro and Micro Nutrients: How Should It Be Adjusted?

The Importance of Micronutrients: Vitamins, Minerals, Antioxidants

Micronutrients are nutrients such as vitamins, minerals, and antioxidants that are essential for the healthy functioning of the body but need to be consumed in only small amounts. These micronutrients support the body's metabolism, strengthen the immune system, and provide protection against various diseases. Below, the main components of micronutrients and their effects on health are detailed.

1. **Vitamins** Vitamins are organic compounds that support various functions in the body and are generally divided into two groups:
   - **Fat-Soluble Vitamins:** Vitamins A, D, E, and K can be found in fatty foods because they are soluble in fat and can be stored in the body. These vitamins play crucial roles in enhancing the immune system, supporting cell health, and contributing to bone health.
   - **Water-Soluble Vitamins:** Vitamins that dissolve in water, such as vitamin C and the B vitamins, cannot be stored in the body and must be consumed regularly. These vitamins are essential for energy production, nervous system health, and immune function (Hoffman et al., 2013).

Benefits:

- Vitamins play a significant role in metabolic processes and act as coenzymes for many biochemical reactions.
- They enhance the immune system, increasing resistance to diseases.
- They improve skin and eye health and elevate energy levels.

2. **Minerals** Minerals are inorganic compounds that serve many important functions in the body. The essential minerals required by the body include:
   - **Macrominerals:** Minerals such as calcium, phosphorus, potassium, magnesium, sodium, and chloride are found in large amounts in the body and have significant functions. For example, calcium is critical for bone health (Weaver, 2013).
   - **Trace Elements:** Minerals like iron, zinc, copper, manganese, iodine, and selenium are present in smaller amounts but perform vital functions. For example, iron is necessary for hemoglobin, which carries oxygen.

Benefits:

- Minerals regulate cellular functions and contribute to enzyme activation.
- They help maintain electrolyte balance and fluid balance.

- They are essential for muscle function and nerve transmission.
3. **Antioxidants** Antioxidants are compounds that protect cells from oxidative stress by combating free radicals. Many vitamins and minerals found in nature exhibit antioxidant properties. Key antioxidants include:
    - **Vitamin C:** Soluble in water and plays many vital roles in the body, particularly for immune system and skin health.
    - **Vitamin E:** A fat-soluble vitamin that protects cell membranes and supports skin health.
    - **Selenium:** This trace element supports the function of antioxidant enzymes and helps strengthen the immune system (Rayman, 2012).

Benefits:

- Protects cell health by reducing the effects of oxidative stress.
- May lower the risk of chronic diseases, cancers, and age-related illnesses.
- Enhances the immune system, increasing resistance to diseases.

Micronutrients are vital for a healthy life. Vitamins, minerals, and antioxidants regulate the body's metabolism, support the immune system, and create positive effects on overall health. A balanced and varied diet is necessary to ensure adequate intake of these micronutrients. Foods rich in micronutrients, such as fruits, vegetables, whole grains, nuts, and legumes, form the foundation of a healthy diet. Therefore, developing healthy eating habits to increase micronutrient intake is a critical step for overall health and well-being.

Flexibility and Sustainability in Nutrition Programs

Nutrition programs help individuals adopt a healthy lifestyle, with flexibility and sustainability as key elements. A flexible and sustainable approach to nutrition provides positive effects on both physical and psychological health, facilitating individuals' long-term goals.

1. **Flexibility** Flexibility in nutrition programs allows individuals to be open to different food options and make healthy choices without strict dietary restrictions. Several key elements of a flexible nutrition approach include:
    - **Variety:** Including a variety of foods in the nutrition program is essential for obtaining all necessary nutrients. Vegetables and fruits of different colors, whole grains, and protein sources create a nutritionally rich diet (López-Olmeda et al., 2020).
    - **Emotional and Social Eating:** Meals are a part of social interactions and emotional experiences. A flexible nutrition approach allows individuals to enjoy delicious foods on special occasions or in social settings while helping them maintain their healthy habits (Davis et al., 2016).

- **Individual Preferences and Needs:** Each individual has different nutritional needs and preferences. A flexible approach enables individuals to develop a personalized nutrition program tailored to their needs, allowing them to stay healthy sustainably.

2. **Sustainability** A sustainable nutrition program helps meet individual health needs while minimizing environmental impacts. Components of a sustainable diet include:
    - **Local and Seasonal Foods:** Consuming local and seasonal products reduces the environmental impact of the food system and enhances the freshness of food. Foods consumed in season are often more nutritious and flavorful (Smith et al., 2014).
    - **Plant-Based Nutrition:** Making plant-based foods (vegetables, fruits, legumes, grains) the foundation of the diet is essential for environmental sustainability. Plant-based foods are associated with lower greenhouse gas emissions compared to animal-based foods and reduce ecological footprints (Willett et al., 2019).
    - **Reducing Food Waste:** A sustainable nutrition program includes strategies to minimize food waste. By shopping with a plan and utilizing leftover food, both economic and environmental benefits can be achieved.

3. **Creating a Flexible and Sustainable Nutrition Program** To create a flexible and sustainable nutrition program, the following steps can be taken:
    - **Goal Setting:** Identifying personal health goals is the first step in creating a sustainable diet. Goals such as weight loss, increasing energy, or improving overall health can guide appropriate food choices.
    - **Planning and Preparation:** Creating weekly meal plans promotes the consumption of healthy and diverse foods. Preparing in advance makes it easier to find healthy alternatives to unhealthy snacks.
    - **Mindful Eating:** Understanding how emotional and social factors affect eating supports a flexible nutrition approach. Individuals can better manage their eating habits and preferences.
    - **Environmental Awareness:** Prioritizing local and sustainable food sources while considering the environmental impact of the nutrition program contributes not only to a healthy diet but also to the protection of the planet.

Flexibility and sustainability are fundamental components of nutrition programs. These elements facilitate individuals' adoption of healthy eating habits while also reducing environmental impacts. Establishing a healthy and balanced diet improves individuals' overall health and represents an important step towards environmental sustainability. Therefore, adopting flexible and sustainable approaches in nutrition programs helps maintain a healthy lifestyle sustainably.

The Role of Complex and Simple Carbohydrates

Carbohydrates are essential nutrients that serve as the body's energy source. The carbohydrates in our diet can be divided into two main groups based on their structure: simple and complex. While both types provide energy, they perform different roles in the body and have varying effects on health. Here is a detailed examination of the role of complex and simple carbohydrates:

1. **Simple Carbohydrates**

Simple carbohydrates consist of one or two sugar units in their molecular structure. They are digested quickly and can be used rapidly as an energy source. Simple carbohydrates include:

- **Monosaccharides:** Simple sugars such as glucose, fructose, and galactose. Glucose is the body's primary energy source.
- **Disaccharides:** Formed by the combination of two monosaccharides, such as sucrose (table sugar), lactose (milk sugar), and maltose.

1.1. **Role and Effects**

- **Rapid Energy Supply:** Simple carbohydrates quickly raise blood sugar levels, providing immediate energy. Consuming them before sports or intense physical activities can boost energy levels.
- **Effect on Satiety:** Excessive consumption of simple carbohydrates can cause rapid spikes and subsequent drops in blood sugar. These fluctuations can negatively impact the feeling of fullness, increasing hunger (Zhao et al., 2015).
- **Insulin Response:** The rapid absorption of simple carbohydrates leads to increased insulin levels. Continuous high insulin levels can increase the risk of insulin resistance and metabolic syndrome (Cohen et al., 2012).

2. **Complex Carbohydrates**

Complex carbohydrates consist of more complex structures made up of three or more sugar units. These carbohydrates are rich in fiber, vitamins, and minerals. Complex carbohydrates include:

- **Starch:** Found in potatoes, rice, corn, and grains.
- **Fiber:** Abundant in vegetables, fruits, whole grains, and legumes.

2.1. **Role and Effects**

- **Sustained Energy Supply:** Because complex carbohydrates take longer to digest, they provide a slower release of energy. This results in long-lasting energy and supports a stable increase in blood sugar (Slavin, 2005).
- **Feeling of Fullness:** Fiber-rich complex carbohydrates remain in the digestive system longer, enhancing the feeling of fullness. This can help with weight control.

- **Digestive Health:** Fiber contributes to healthy digestive system function. It regulates bowel movements and helps prevent digestive issues such as constipation (Anderson et al., 2009).
- **Support for Metabolism:** Since complex carbohydrates are nutrient-rich foods, they have positive effects on overall health and metabolism.

3. **Balanced Consumption of Simple and Complex Carbohydrates**

A balanced diet requires an appropriate amount of both simple and complex carbohydrates. Here are some tips for healthy eating:

- **Limiting Simple Carbohydrates:** It is important to avoid processed foods that contain refined sugars and to prefer simple sugars from natural fruits and vegetables.
- **Choosing Complex Carbohydrates:** The consumption of fiber-rich foods like whole grains, legumes, and vegetables should be increased.
- **Balanced Nutrition:** In addition to carbohydrates, protein and healthy fats should also be part of a balanced diet. This helps balance energy levels and supports overall health.

Both simple and complex carbohydrates perform essential functions for the body. Simple carbohydrates provide quick energy, while complex carbohydrates offer long-lasting energy and satiety. A balanced consumption of these two types of carbohydrates in a healthy diet supports metabolism and positively affects overall health. Choosing the right carbohydrate sources is one of the cornerstones of a healthy lifestyle.

Considerations for Meeting Vitamin and Mineral Needs

Vitamins and minerals are critical micronutrients necessary for the healthy functioning of the body. Each serves different biological functions and supports various systems in the body. Meeting vitamin and mineral needs is essential for overall health and well-being. Here are important points to consider for meeting vitamin and mineral needs:

1. **Diversifying Food Sources**
- **Consuming Different Food Groups:** To meet vitamin and mineral needs, it is important to consume a balanced variety of food groups, including vegetables, fruits, whole grains, dairy products, meat, fish, and legumes. Each food group offers different sources of vitamins and minerals. For example, dark green leafy vegetables are rich in vitamin K and iron, while dairy products provide calcium and vitamin D (Weaver et al., 2016).
- **Colorful Vegetables and Fruits:** Colorful fruits and vegetables offer different vitamin and mineral contents. For example, orange fruits are rich in beta-carotene (a precursor to vitamin A), red vegetables contain lycopene, and purple fruits have antioxidant

properties. Choosing a variety of colors allows for a wider range of nutrients (Slavin & Lloyd, 2012).

2. **Avoiding Processed Foods**
- **Limiting Refined and Processed Foods:** Processed foods are often low in vitamin and mineral content and contain added sugars and unhealthy fats. Preferring natural and fresh foods can increase vitamin and mineral intake.
- **Reading Labels:** Reading food labels is essential for understanding content and making healthy choices. Avoiding products high in added sugars, salt, and saturated fats can improve nutritional quality.

3. **Supplement Use**
- **Nutritional Supplements:** If adequate amounts of vitamins and minerals cannot be obtained from a balanced diet, food supplements may be used with doctor advice. Certain situations, such as pregnancy, breastfeeding, aging, or specific health conditions, may increase the need for certain vitamins and minerals (Nascimento et al., 2017).
- **Balanced Use:** Excessive use of supplements can lead to toxic effects from certain vitamins and minerals. Therefore, caution should be exercised in the use of supplements, and consulting a health professional when needed is recommended.

4. **Bioavailability**
- **Food Preparation:** Proper preparation of foods is important for preserving vitamin and mineral content. For example, overcooking vegetables can lead to loss of some vitamins. Methods like steaming or consuming raw can help maintain nutritional value (Wang et al., 2016).
- **Supporting Absorption:** Some vitamins require fat for absorption. For example, vitamins A, D, E, and K are fat-soluble vitamins. Therefore, adding olive oil to vegetable salads can enhance vitamin absorption (Havala et al., 2016).

5. **Lifestyle and Habits**
- **Regular Eating:** Regular and balanced eating habits help meet vitamin and mineral needs. Skipping meals can negatively affect nutrient intake.
- **Water Consumption:** Adequate water intake is necessary for transporting and absorbing nutrients in the body. Water also helps eliminate toxins from the body.

- **Physical Activity:** Regular physical activity allows the body to use nutrients more efficiently and improves overall health. Exercise can influence the need for vitamins and minerals by increasing metabolic rate (Fitzgerald et al., 2016).

Meeting vitamin and mineral needs is essential for maintaining a healthy lifestyle. Diversifying food sources, avoiding processed foods, using supplements when necessary, enhancing bioavailability, and adopting healthy lifestyle habits can support vitamin and mineral intake, improving overall health. A healthy diet and lifestyle play a crucial role in effectively meeting the body's micronutrient requirements.

5. Nutrition Strategies That Support Fat Burning

Intermittent Fasting and Its Effects on Fat Burning

Intermittent fasting is a dietary pattern that combines eating and fasting periods within a specific timeframe. This method has gained popularity in recent years and has been the subject of many studies. Intermittent fasting practices are generally seen as strategies believed to have positive effects on weight loss, fat burning, and overall health. Here's a comprehensive review of intermittent fasting and its effects on fat burning:

1. **Definition and Methods of Intermittent Fasting**
   Intermittent fasting can be implemented in several different ways. The most common methods are:
   - **16/8 Method**: Fasting for 16 hours of the day and eating during an 8-hour window. For example, eating is allowed between noon and 8 PM.
   - **5:2 Diet**: Normal eating for 5 days of the week, while calorie intake is limited to 500-600 calories on 2 days.
   - **Alternate Day Fasting**: Fasting for a specific period each day (e.g., 24 hours) while eating normally on other days.
     These methods can help individuals change their eating habits and limit calorie intake.
2. **Mechanisms Supporting Fat Burning**
   Intermittent fasting can trigger several biological mechanisms that support fat burning:
   - **Decreased Insulin Levels**: During intermittent fasting, insulin levels drop between eating periods. Low insulin levels reduce fat storage and increase fat burning. Insulin promotes the storage of fat in fat cells; thus, a decrease in insulin facilitates the use of fats as an energy source (Patterson & Sears, 2017).

- o **Increase in Growth Hormone**: Intermittent fasting practices can lead to an increase in growth hormone (HGH) levels. HGH is a hormone that promotes fat burning and helps maintain muscle mass. High levels of growth hormone support the body's ability to burn fats and preserve muscles (Ho et al., 1988).
- o **Increased Autophagy**: Autophagy is the process by which cells repair themselves. Intermittent fasting can stimulate this process, promote cellular repair, and lead to anti-aging effects. Autophagy helps eliminate toxins and damaged components accumulated in cells (Levine et al., 2017).

3. **Research on Its Effects on Fat Burning**

Various studies have examined the effects of intermittent fasting practices on fat loss:

- o **Weight Loss**: Many studies have observed that individuals practicing intermittent fasting experience more significant weight loss compared to those on traditional diet programs. Particularly, regularly practiced methods like the 16/8 method have been found effective against obesity and overweight (Varady & Hellerstein, 2009).
- o **Body Composition**: Intermittent fasting can reduce fat mass while helping to maintain muscle mass. Research indicates that intermittent fasting practices significantly decrease body fat percentage while preserving muscle mass (Moro et al., 2016).

4. **Other Health Benefits**

Intermittent fasting not only supports fat burning but also offers various health benefits:

- o **Metabolic Health**: Intermittent fasting improves insulin levels and may reduce insulin resistance, thereby lowering the risk of type 2 diabetes (Trepanowski & Bloomer, 2010).
- o **Heart Health**: Studies show that intermittent fasting practices can reduce cholesterol and triglyceride levels, which decreases the risk of heart diseases (Klempel et al., 2013).
- o **Brain Health**: Intermittent fasting may help increase neurological factors that support brain health. It is believed to elevate levels of BDNF (brain-derived neurotrophic factor), which protects brain health (Mattson et al., 2017).

5. **Considerations**

It is important to remember that intermittent fasting practices may not be suitable for everyone. Caution should be exercised in the following situations:

- o **Health Issues**: Individuals with diabetes, eating disorders, or chronic illnesses should consult a healthcare professional before practicing intermittent fasting.
- o **Pregnancy and Breastfeeding**: Adequate and balanced nutrient intake is essential during pregnancy and breastfeeding; thus, intermittent fasting practices may not be recommended.

- **Individual Differences**: Each individual has a different body composition, metabolic rate, and lifestyle. While intermittent fasting may be effective for some, it may not yield the same results for others.

Intermittent fasting stands out as an effective dietary strategy supporting fat burning. Mechanisms such as decreased insulin levels, increased growth hormone, and the triggering of cellular repair processes promote fat loss. However, it should be noted that intermittent fasting practices may not be suitable for everyone and should be applied with consideration of health status. For the best results, intermittent fasting can be most effective when combined with a balanced diet and regular physical activity.

Carbohydrate Cycling and Low-Carbohydrate Diets

Carbohydrate cycling is a dietary strategy aimed at improving body composition by regulating the intake of different amounts of carbohydrates on specific days or periods. Low-carbohydrate diets are those in which a significant portion of the total daily calorie intake comes from protein and fats rather than carbohydrates. Both approaches are used for goals such as weight loss, fat burning, and preserving muscle mass. Here's a comprehensive review of carbohydrate cycling and low-carbohydrate diets:

1. **Definition and Methods of Carbohydrate Cycling**

   Carbohydrate cycling typically involves creating a dietary pattern that includes both high and low carbohydrate days. This method is implemented to enhance muscle glycogen stores and promote fat burning. The fundamental methods of carbohydrate cycling include:

   - **High Carbohydrate Days**: Increasing carbohydrate intake on specific days of the week to replenish muscle glycogen stores and revitalize metabolism. These days are typically aligned with intense training days.
   - **Low Carbohydrate Days**: Reducing carbohydrate intake on other days to increase fat burning. These days may be associated with rest or light training days.
   - **Cyclic Programs**: Carbohydrate cycling is repeated within a specific cycle, for example, implementing 3 high carbohydrate days and 4 low carbohydrate days per week.

2. **Definition of Low-Carbohydrate Diets**

   Low-carbohydrate diets are those in which 10-30% of total daily calorie intake comes from carbohydrates, while the remainder comes from protein and fats. The key features of these diets are:

   - **Carbohydrate Restriction**: Carbohydrate intake is typically limited to between 20-100 grams. This amount can vary based on the type of diet.
   - **Emphasis on Protein and Fats**: Protein and healthy fats are prominent in low-carbohydrate diets. This can increase satiety and promote fat burning.

- **Ketogenic Diet**: A type of low-carbohydrate diet that induces a state of ketosis in the body. In this state, fats are used as an energy source.

3. **Effects of Carbohydrate Cycling and Low-Carbohydrate Diets**
   - **Weight Loss and Fat Burning**: Research suggests that low-carbohydrate diets and carbohydrate cycling can be effective in weight loss and fat burning. Low carbohydrate intake decreases insulin levels, reduces fat storage, and promotes the use of fat as an energy source (Glynn et al., 2013).
   - **Increased Fat Burning**: Carbohydrate cycling allows the body to both burn fat and preserve muscle mass. High carbohydrate days can enhance training performance by replenishing muscle glycogen stores, while low carbohydrate days promote fat burning (Varady & Hellerstein, 2009).
   - **Metabolic Effects**: Low-carbohydrate diets and carbohydrate cycling can positively affect metabolism. Studies show that low carbohydrate intake can increase metabolic rate and reduce insulin resistance (Krebs-Smith et al., 2010).
   - **Energy Balance**: Carbohydrate cycling can positively impact the body's energy balance. Increased energy intake on high carbohydrate days can support muscle development (Moro et al., 2016).

4. **Considerations**

   While carbohydrate cycling and low-carbohydrate diets may be beneficial for some individuals, they can also pose challenges for others. The following points should be considered:
   - **Individual Differences**: Each person's metabolism, activity level, and health status differ. Therefore, it is essential to tailor these diets to the individual.
   - **Long-Term Sustainability**: Low-carbohydrate diets and carbohydrate cycling may be challenging for some individuals. Establishing a sustainable diet plan in the long term is essential for developing healthy lifestyle habits.
   - **Nutritional Value**: In low-carbohydrate diets, healthy fats and protein sources should be chosen. Adequate intake of vitamins and minerals is also crucial, making vegetable and fruit consumption important.

Carbohydrate cycling and low-carbohydrate diets can be effective strategies for weight loss and fat burning. Both approaches can help individuals change their eating habits and maintain a healthy lifestyle. However, it is essential that these diets are tailored to individual needs and combined with a balanced dietary regimen to achieve the best results. Especially in terms of long-term health and sustainability, developing healthy lifestyle habits is critical.

Smart Snacks: Consumption at the Right Time and Amount

Snacks hold an important place in a healthy eating regimen. However, snacks consumed in the right type and amount, referred to as smart snacks, not only satisfy hunger but also boost energy levels, enhance focus, and support overall health. This section will provide detailed information about what smart snacks are and how to consume them at the right time and in the right amounts.

1. **What Are Smart Snacks?**

   Smart snacks are foods that are high in nutritional value, containing balanced components, and are typically unprocessed or minimally processed. These snacks include healthy fats, protein, and fiber. Smart snacks should be preferred over unhealthy alternatives. Examples include:

- Nuts (almonds, walnuts, hazelnuts)
- Fresh fruits (apple, pear, strawberry)
- Yogurt or strained yogurt
- Hummus and vegetables
- Whole grain crackers or rice cakes

2. **Consumption at the Right Times**

   Consuming smart snacks at the right time can enhance both physical and mental performance. Here are the best times for snack consumption:

2.1. Between Meals

Snacking between main meals is ideal for balancing blood sugar levels and controlling hunger. Especially during intense working hours or before and after workouts, smart snacks should be preferred.

2.2. When Energy Levels Drop

When energy levels drop in the middle of the day, having a healthy snack can help alleviate fatigue and increase concentration. For example, a handful of nuts or a piece of fruit consumed after lunch can boost your energy levels.

2.3. Before and After Exercise

Snacks rich in carbohydrates and protein consumed before exercise can enhance performance, while protein sources consumed after exercise support muscle repair. For instance, a banana and yogurt can speed up the recovery process after a workout.

3. **Consumption in the Right Amounts**

   The amount of snacks varies depending on the overall dietary plan and individual needs. Below are general guidelines for the right amounts:

3.1. Portion Control

Portion control of smart snacks is critical to prevent excessive calorie intake. In general:

- Nuts: 30 grams (about a handful)
- Fruits: 1 medium-sized fruit or 1 cup of fresh fruit
- Yogurt: 150-200 grams

- Hummus: 2-4 tablespoons with 1 cup of vegetables

3.2. Individual Needs

The amount of snacks can vary based on an individual's age, gender, level of physical activity, and health status. Active individuals may consume more snacks due to higher energy needs, while less active individuals may need to reduce their intake.

4. Considerations When Choosing Smart Snacks

- **Nutritional Value:** The chosen snacks should be high in nutritional value. Avoid processed foods and opt for natural, nourishing sources.
- **Sugar Content:** Options without added sugar or low in sugar should be preferred. Sugary snacks can cause sudden energy spikes followed by crashes.
- **Fiber and Protein:** Snacks rich in fiber and protein help you feel fuller for a longer time.

Smart snacks are an important part of a healthy lifestyle. When consumed at the right time and in the right amounts, these snacks not only help control hunger but also boost energy levels and support overall health. Choosing nutritious snacks tailored to individual needs offers an effective strategy for achieving healthy living goals. By incorporating healthy snacks into your daily routine, you can establish a balanced eating regimen and improve your health.

Frequent Meals or Long Intervals? Advantages and Disadvantages

Eating habits have a significant impact on individual health and quality of life. The choice between frequent meals and long intervals can affect weight control, energy levels, and overall health. This section will address the advantages and disadvantages of both approaches.

1. Frequent Meals

Definition: Frequent meals involve consuming 5-6 small meals per day. This approach aims to reduce feelings of hunger and stabilize blood sugar levels.

1.1. Advantages

- **Maintaining Blood Sugar Balance:** Eating frequently can help maintain stable blood sugar levels. This is particularly beneficial for individuals with insulin resistance or diabetes (Schafer et al., 2018).
- **Hunger Control:** Frequent meals reduce feelings of hunger, thereby decreasing the risk of overeating. This can be a positive factor for weight control (Moro et al., 2016).
- **Metabolism Rate:** Regular meals can keep metabolism active. However, the degree of this effect may vary from person to person (Jakubowicz et al., 2013).
- **Energy Levels:** Eating regularly throughout the day can help keep energy levels more stable.

1.2. Disadvantages

- **Time Management:** Eating frequently can be time-consuming for some individuals. It can be challenging for those with a busy lifestyle.
- **Excess Calorie Intake:** If poor choices are made, frequent meals can increase total calorie intake, potentially leading to weight gain (Kleiner et al., 2018).
- **Digestive Issues:** Some individuals may report that constant eating can strain the digestive system.

2. **Long Intervals**

   Definition: Long intervals involve eating 2-3 main meals per day. In this approach, there are longer periods between meals.

2.1. Advantages

- **Digestive Time:** Long intervals give the digestive system a rest. This can improve digestive health for some individuals (Gonzalez et al., 2018).
- **Time Savings:** Cooking and eating less frequently can be advantageous in terms of time management. It offers a practical option, especially for busy individuals.
- **Weight Control:** Some studies suggest that eating less frequently can reduce total calorie intake and support weight loss (Varady & Hellerstein, 2009).

2.2. Disadvantages

- **Hunger Feelings:** Going long periods without food can increase feelings of hunger. This may lead to a risk of overeating and unhealthy food choices.
- **Blood Sugar Instability:** Long intervals can cause fluctuations in blood sugar levels, potentially leading to energy drops and fatigue (Schafer et al., 2018).
- **Nutritional Deficiencies:** Fewer meals may require careful planning to ensure sufficient nutrient intake. It can be challenging to ensure adequate vitamin and mineral intake.

3. **Which Method Is More Suitable?**

   Both dietary approaches have advantages and disadvantages. The most suitable method depends on factors such as an individual's lifestyle, metabolism, health status, and personal preferences. The key is to create a balanced diet and develop a nutrition plan tailored to individual needs.

When choosing between frequent meals and long intervals, it is important for individuals to consider their own lifestyles, goals, and health conditions. There are situations where both approaches can be effective, and the best results can be achieved with a personalized plan. Maintaining healthy eating habits and implementing a balanced diet play a critical role in enhancing overall health and quality of life.

6. Boosting Metabolism: Food Choices and Lifestyle

Foods and Drinks That Accelerate Metabolism

Metabolism is the process by which the body produces and expends energy. Increasing metabolic rate can aid in weight control, elevate energy levels, and have positive effects on overall health. Some foods and drinks contain components with the potential to accelerate metabolism. This section will explore the most effective foods and drinks that support metabolism.

1. **Green Tea** Green tea can speed up metabolism due to its caffeine and antioxidants (especially catechins). Research has shown that green tea increases fat oxidation and boosts energy expenditure (Hursel et al., 2009). Consuming several cups of green tea a day can support calorie burning.
2. **Caffeine** Caffeine is one of the most popular substances for boosting metabolism. Caffeinated beverages like coffee, tea, and some energy drinks can accelerate metabolism in the short term. Caffeine can enhance physical performance and promote fat burning (Acheson et al., 2004). However, it's important to avoid excessive caffeine consumption.
3. **Spices** Spices contain natural components that have the potential to increase metabolism, especially:
- **Red Pepper**: Contains capsaicin, which can speed up metabolism. Research shows that red pepper increases calorie expenditure (Ludy et al., 2012).
- **Ginger**: Aids digestion and can boost metabolic rate. Ginger tea or its use in meals is recommended.
4. **Protein Sources** Protein requires more energy to digest. High-protein foods can increase metabolism due to their thermal effect. High-protein foods include:
- Chicken, turkey, fish
- Eggs
- Dairy products (yogurt, cheese)
- Legumes (lentils, chickpeas)
5. **Water** Adequate water intake is vital for the proper functioning of metabolism. Studies have shown that drinking cold water can temporarily boost metabolism. The body expends energy to heat cold water (Boschmann et al., 2003). Daily water consumption is important for enhancing metabolic rate.
6. **Whole Grains** Whole grains are rich in fiber. Fiber slows digestion, helping you feel full longer. Whole grains also contain B vitamins that support metabolism. Examples include:
- Oats
- Brown rice
- Whole wheat bread
7. **Apple Cider Vinegar** Apple cider vinegar has been studied for its potential positive effects on metabolism. It may help balance blood sugar levels and increase fat burning. However, it should be consumed diluted with water to avoid excessive intake (Kondo et al., 2009).

8. **Yogurt and Probiotics** Yogurt and other probiotic sources can positively affect metabolism by supporting gut health. A healthy gut flora aids the efficient functioning of the digestive system and can enhance nutrient absorption.
9. **Dark Chocolate** Dark chocolate can accelerate metabolism due to its flavonoid content. However, care should be taken regarding its sugar and fat content. Dark chocolate with 70% or higher cocoa content is recommended.

Foods and drinks that accelerate metabolism are an essential part of a healthy lifestyle. Regular exercise, in conjunction with a balanced diet, is critical for increasing metabolic rate and supporting overall health. By incorporating these foods and drinks into your nutrition plan, you can boost your energy levels and achieve your weight control goals. However, consuming just these foods is not sufficient for adopting a healthy lifestyle; regular physical activity and adequate sleep are also important.

The Effect of Water Consumption on Fat Burning

Water is a vital component for life and plays a critical role in many bodily functions. Its effects on fat burning and weight control are fundamental to a healthy lifestyle. This section will detail the effects of water consumption on fat burning.

1. **Accelerating Metabolism** Water can increase metabolic rate. Research has shown that water temporarily boosts energy expenditure. For example, drinking water has been found to increase calorie burning by helping to regulate body temperature. One study observed that drinking 500 ml of water increased metabolism by about 30% (Boschmann et al., 2003). This effect is related to the role of water in the digestive system and the body's cooling mechanisms.
2. **Promoting Satiety** Water can increase the feeling of fullness, reducing the risk of overeating. Drinking water before meals enhances the feeling of fullness in the stomach, leading to a reduced need to eat more. Studies have shown that water consumption is particularly effective in reducing calorie intake (Stookey et al., 2008). Adequate water intake helps control hunger, supporting healthy eating habits.
3. **Fat Oxidation** Adequate water intake supports fat oxidation. The body needs water during the process of converting fats into energy. Water deficiency can negatively affect the efficiency of fat burning. Additionally, water plays an important role in the metabolism of fatty acids and energy production in cells (Maughan & Burke, 2012). Thus, sufficient water intake can increase fat burning.
4. **Fluid Balance and Exercise Performance** Sufficient fluid intake during exercise enhances performance and supports fat burning. Water regulates body temperature, increasing endurance during exercise. Additionally, dehydration can lower energy levels and negatively affect performance (Gonzalez-Alonso et al., 1999). Ensuring adequate

water consumption before, during, and after exercise is an effective strategy for supporting fat burning.

5. **Water Consumption and Strategies for Fat Burning**

- **Setting Daily Water Goals**: Personal water needs vary based on age, gender, activity level, and climate conditions. A general recommendation is to drink at least 2-3 liters of water daily.
- **Drinking Water Before Meals**: Drinking a glass of water 30 minutes before meals can enhance the feeling of fullness and reduce overall calorie intake.
- **Water Consumption Before and After Exercise**: Paying attention to water intake before, during, and after exercise improves performance and supports fat burning.

Water consumption is an important factor supporting fat burning. Its effects, such as accelerating metabolism, promoting satiety, increasing fat oxidation, and improving exercise performance, contribute to maintaining a healthy lifestyle. Ensuring adequate water intake is a critical strategy for achieving weight control goals. Increasing water consumption can improve not only fat burning but also overall health.

Stress Management, Sleep Regulation, and Rest

Stress management, sleep regulation, and rest are essential components of a healthy lifestyle. These three factors have a significant impact on physical health, mental balance, and overall quality of life. This section will examine stress management techniques, the importance of sleep regulation, and the benefits of rest.

1. **Stress Management**

Stress is an inevitable part of daily life, but if not managed effectively, it can negatively impact physical and mental health. Stress management involves identifying the sources of stress, coping with these sources, and developing strategies to deal with stress. Stress management techniques include:

- **Relaxation of Mind and Body**: Meditation, yoga, and deep breathing exercises provide mental and physical relaxation. Research has shown that these techniques can reduce stress levels (Goyal et al., 2014).
- **Time Management**: Planning and prioritizing daily tasks can help manage stress. Good time management reduces the sense of urgency and allows for more efficient completion of tasks.
- **Physical Activity**: Exercise releases endorphins and is an effective method for coping with stress. Regular physical activity reduces the negative effects of stress and improves overall mood (Mikkelsen et al., 2017).

- **Social Support**: Communicating with family and friends and receiving emotional support facilitates coping with stress. Social support systems play an important role in managing stress.

2. **Sleep Regulation**

Sleep is a vital process for the body's renewal, improvement of mental functions, and maintenance of overall health. Getting sufficient and quality sleep has positive effects on stress management and mood:

- **Sleep Needs**: Adults are generally recommended to sleep 7-9 hours a day. Adequate sleep strengthens the immune system, regulates metabolism, and improves mood (Hirshkowitz et al., 2015).
- **Sleep Hygiene**: Attention to sleep hygiene is important for improving sleep quality. This includes establishing a regular sleep schedule, creating a comfortable sleep environment, and limiting the use of electronic devices.
- **Stress and Sleep**: High levels of stress can negatively affect sleep quality. Implementing stress management techniques can enhance sleep quality. Techniques such as regular exercise, meditation, and deep breathing can facilitate falling asleep (Zhang et al., 2015).

3. **Benefits of Rest**

Rest is necessary for the renewal of the body and mind. Sufficient rest reduces stress levels, increases energy levels, and improves overall health:

- **Physical Rest**: Adequate rest helps repair and strengthen muscles. Resting after exercise enhances performance and reduces the risk of injury.
- **Mental Rest**: Mental rest improves attention and concentration. Taking short breaks can help the mind recharge and work more efficiently.
- **Enhancing Creativity**: Rest can boost creativity. Research indicates that rest contributes to the emergence of new ideas and the development of problem-solving abilities (Kounios & Beeman, 2009).

Stress management, sleep regulation, and rest are fundamental elements for maintaining a healthy life. Effectively managing stress, obtaining adequate sleep, and taking time for rest are important for preserving physical and mental health. The balanced integration of these three factors enhances individuals' overall quality of life and helps them adopt a healthier lifestyle. Therefore, paying attention to these elements in daily life is a critical step toward maintaining a healthy and balanced life.

Activity Level and Supporting with Exercise

Activity level is a term that defines how much individuals move, exercise, and engage in physical activities in their daily lives. An adequate activity level is an important part of a healthy lifestyle and plays a crucial role, especially in supporting fat burning. This section will address the importance of activity level, the benefits of exercise, and ways to create a lifestyle supported by exercise.

1. **Importance of Activity Level**

Activity level directly affects individuals' health. Physical activity has positive effects on cardiovascular health, metabolism, and psychological well-being:

- **Heart Health**: Regular physical activity reduces the risk of heart disease. Exercise strengthens the heart muscle and improves blood circulation (Myers et al., 2002).
- **Metabolism**: Physical activity helps accelerate metabolism. Adequate activity increases fat burning and improves insulin sensitivity (Bock et al., 2015).
- **Mental Health**: Exercise releases endorphins, which improve mood and reduce stress levels. Regular activity can alleviate symptoms of depression and anxiety (Craft & Perna, 2004).

2. **Benefits of Exercise**

Exercise has numerous positive effects on both physical and mental health. Some benefits of exercise include:

- **Supporting Fat Burning**: Exercise supports fat burning by increasing calorie expenditure. Aerobic exercises (running, cycling) and resistance training (weight lifting) are effective for increasing fat loss (Willis et al., 2012).
- **Muscle Development**: Resistance exercises increase muscle mass and elevate the metabolic rate at rest. More muscle mass leads to more calorie burning while at rest (Phillips & Van Loon, 2011).
- **Increased Endurance and Strength**: Regular exercise enhances physical endurance and improves overall strength. This helps individuals perform daily activities more easily and effectively.

3. **Creating an Exercise-Supported Lifestyle**

Incorporating exercise and physical activity into your daily routine is essential for building a balanced lifestyle. Here are some suggestions to support this process:

- **Setting Goals**: Setting realistic and achievable goals increases motivation. When defining your goals, ensure they meet SMART (Specific, Measurable, Achievable, Relevant, Time-bound) criteria.
- **Creating an Exercise Program**: It is recommended to engage in at least 150 minutes of moderate-intensity aerobic activity or 75 minutes of high-intensity activity each week. Additionally, incorporating resistance training twice a week is also important (U.S. Department of Health and Human Services, 2018).

- **Staying Active in Daily Life**: Making changes to be more active in daily life, such as using stairs instead of elevators, going for walks, and engaging in active hobbies, can be beneficial.
- **Making Exercise Fun**: Making your exercises enjoyable increases sustainability. Social and fun activities, such as dancing, team sports, or hiking, can be preferred.

Activity level and exercise are fundamental components of a healthy lifestyle. Adequate physical activity supports fat burning while enhancing overall health and quality of life. Exercise positively affects not only physical but also mental health. Therefore, it is important for individuals to increase their activity levels and engage in regular exercise in their daily lives. Adopting a healthy lifestyle improves quality of life, allowing individuals to feel more energetic, happier, and healthier.

7. Exercise and Fat Burning

The Impact of Cardio and Resistance Training on Fat Burning

Cardio (aerobic) and resistance (weight) training are essential components of a healthy lifestyle. While both types of training support fat burning, they also have positive effects on the body's overall health and physical performance. This section will provide information on the roles of cardio and resistance training in fat burning and how they can be effectively utilized.

1. **The Impact of Cardio Training on Fat Burning**

Cardio workouts are physical activities that promote calorie burning by increasing heart rate. Aerobic exercises typically include activities performed for extended periods at low to moderate intensity. The effects of cardio training on fat burning include:

- **Calorie Burning:** Cardio workouts increase calorie expenditure during and after exercise. High-Intensity Interval Training (HIIT) can particularly help burn more calories in a shorter time (Gibala et al., 2014).
- **Fat Oxidation:** Cardio exercises enhance fat oxidation, helping the body use energy sources more effectively. Long-duration aerobic exercises are especially effective in increasing fat burning (Achten & Jeukendrup, 2004).
- **Cardiovascular Health:** Cardio training improves heart and vascular health. Improved heart health supports overall well-being and helps speed up metabolism in individuals who exercise regularly (Thyfault & Booth, 2011).

2. **The Impact of Resistance Training on Fat Burning**

Resistance training consists of weightlifting or resistance exercises aimed at increasing muscle strength and developing muscle mass. The effects of resistance training on fat burning include:

- **Increase in Muscle Mass:** Resistance training increases muscle mass, thereby raising the basal metabolic rate. More muscle mass causes the body to burn more calories at rest (Coyle, 2002).
- **Sustained Fat Burning:** Resistance training can increase calorie burning in the post-exercise period. This phenomenon is known as "afterburn" (EPOC - Excess Post-exercise Oxygen Consumption). The body supports fat burning by expending more energy after exercise (Hickner et al., 2009).
- **Balanced Body Composition:** Resistance training creates a healthy body composition by maintaining a balance between muscle and fat. This increases fat burning and improves overall health (Ronnestad et al., 2016).

3. **Combined Use of Cardio and Resistance Training**

Combining cardio and resistance training is one of the most effective approaches for supporting fat burning and overall health. Some strategies for integrating the two types of training include:

- **Combined Training Programs:** Engaging in cardio at least three days a week and resistance training two days a week increases fat burning and improves body composition. This combination enables more efficient metabolism.
- **Exercise Variety:** Incorporating different types of exercises (swimming, running, cycling) into both cardio and resistance training diversifies workouts, increases motivation, and helps avoid plateaus.
- **Timing:** The timing between cardio and resistance training may be significant. Some research suggests that performing cardio workouts after resistance training may have more positive effects on muscle mass (Moraes et al., 2017).

Cardio and resistance training play crucial roles in supporting fat burning. While cardio increases calorie burning, resistance training boosts metabolism by increasing muscle mass. Combining these two types of workouts helps individuals reach their fat loss goals while also enhancing overall health and physical performance. It is recommended to create a program that regularly includes both types of training for a healthy lifestyle.

HIIT (High-Intensity Interval Training) and Fat Burning

High-Intensity Interval Training (HIIT) is an effective type of workout that combines short bursts of intense exercise with short rest periods. HIIT is often preferred for fat burning and improving cardiovascular health. This section will examine the effects of HIIT on fat burning, its mechanisms of action, and how it can be implemented.

1. **Effects of HIIT on Fat Burning**

HIIT workouts consist of cycles of short bursts of high-intensity exercise followed by brief low-intensity rest intervals. This structure maximizes calorie burning and maintains fat burning after the workout. The primary effects of HIIT on fat burning are:

- **Increased Calorie Burning:** HIIT workouts lead to greater calorie expenditure than traditional cardio exercises performed for the same duration. Especially short, intense bursts increase energy consumption, supporting fat loss (Laursen & Jenkins, 2002).
- **EPOC (Excess Post-exercise Oxygen Consumption):** HIIT workouts ensure continued calorie burning even after the workout. This phenomenon is known as "EPOC." EPOC increases fat burning due to excess oxygen consumption during the recovery process after exercise (Schoenfeld & Dawes, 2009).
- **Increased Insulin Sensitivity:** HIIT improves insulin sensitivity in muscle cells, allowing for more effective glucose utilization. This helps the body manage energy sources better and reduces fat storage (Babraj et al., 2009).

2. **Mechanisms of HIIT Action**

HIIT creates a series of metabolic and physiological changes in the body. These mechanisms effectively accelerate fat burning and reduce body fat percentage:

- **Increased Hormone Secretion:** HIIT stimulates the secretion of hormones such as growth hormone and norepinephrine, which support fat burning. These hormones act on fat cells to facilitate the use of fats as energy (Boutcher, 2011).
- **Effects on Muscle Fibers:** HIIT activates fast-twitch muscle fibers, helping preserve muscle mass. Maintaining muscle mass supports metabolic rate and accelerates fat burning (Ross & Leveritt, 2001).
- **Metabolic Flexibility:** HIIT enhances the body's ability to utilize different energy sources, such as carbohydrates and fats (metabolic flexibility). This feature allows for more efficient fat burning (Talanian et al., 2007).

3. **Implementing HIIT Workouts**

HIIT can be applied using various types of exercises. While often preferred in cardio-focused workouts like running, cycling, and swimming, it can also be combined with resistance training. Considerations for enhancing the effectiveness of HIIT workouts include:

- **Workout Duration:** HIIT workouts are short but require high intensity. A HIIT workout lasting 15-30 minutes can be effective for fat burning. It's important to adjust the duration according to individual needs.
- **Exercise Selection:** Exercises used in HIIT workouts can be chosen based on personal preference. For instance, 30 seconds of sprinting followed by 30 seconds of rest is an effective HIIT application.

- **Frequency:** Because HIIT workouts are intense, it is not recommended to perform them daily. Doing HIIT 2-3 times a week is sufficient to support fat burning. It is important to include rest days to allow for muscle recovery.

4. **Benefits and Considerations of HIIT Workouts**

While HIIT is highly effective for fat burning, it should be implemented cautiously due to its high-intensity nature:

- **Time Efficiency:** HIIT offers the advantage of maximizing calorie burning in a short time, making it ideal for individuals with time constraints.
- **Muscle Preservation:** There is a risk of muscle loss in intense workouts. It is important to pay attention to adequate protein intake and recovery when practicing HIIT.
- **Injury Risk:** The intense nature of HIIT may increase the risk of injury. Therefore, it is crucial to focus on warm-up and cool-down periods and perform exercises with the correct technique.

HIIT is a powerful tool for fat burning and overall health. It accelerates body metabolism, increases fat oxidation, maximizes calorie burning, and continues fat burning after workouts. It is ideal for individuals with time constraints or those seeking a high-intensity workout. However, due to HIIT's high-intensity nature, it is important to program it appropriately and pay attention to rest intervals.

How to Structure an Exercise Program for Fat Loss

An exercise program designed to support fat loss focuses on increasing the body's energy expenditure while preserving muscle mass. To achieve effective fat loss, it is important to create a balanced program that includes the right types of exercises, intensity, duration, and rest periods. In this section, we will examine how to structure an exercise program that maximizes fat loss.

1. **Types of Exercises and Fat Loss**

   Utilizing different types of exercises when creating an exercise program helps increase fat loss and ensures training variety:

   - **Cardio Exercises:** Cardio (aerobic) exercises increase calorie burning by elevating the heart rate. Exercises such as brisk walking, running, cycling, and swimming support the cardiovascular system while accelerating fat oxidation (Willis et al., 2012).
   - **Resistance Training:** Resistance (weight) training is essential for maintaining and increasing muscle mass. As muscle mass increases, the resting metabolic rate also rises, leading to greater calorie burn in the long term (Strasser et al., 2013). Therefore, it is recommended to engage in resistance training at least 2-3 times a week.
   - **HIIT (High-Intensity Interval Training):** HIIT workouts, which provide high calorie burn in a short period, are an ideal option for accelerating fat loss.

Research shows that HIIT maintains post-workout fat burning due to its short but intense structure (Gibala et al., 2012).

2. **Exercise Intensity and Duration**

Exercise intensity and duration are critical for fat loss. Depending on the structure of the program, the intensity and duration of exercises may vary:

- ○ **Moderate Intensity Cardio:** Performing moderate-intensity cardio 3-4 days a week for 30-45 minutes supports fat loss. Moderate-intensity cardio exercises can be sustained for long periods and improve cardiovascular health.
- ○ **High-Intensity Cardio (Interval Training):** HIIT performed 2-3 days a week for 20-30 minutes increases fat loss in a short time. During intense exercise, the body increases oxygen consumption, triggering the EPOC effect, leading to continued fat burning post-exercise (Schoenfeld, 2010).
- ○ **Resistance Training:** It is recommended to perform resistance training targeting all major muscle groups 2-3 times a week. Performing 3-4 sets with 8-12 repetitions per exercise is ideal. Engaging the muscles supports fat burning while tightening the body.

3. **Rest and Recovery in the Exercise Program**

Rest is a critical component for the sustainability of fat loss and muscle development. The recovery process after intense workouts is important for muscle repair and healthy metabolism:

- ○ **At Least One Rest Day a Week:** At least one rest day should be scheduled per week. This allows the muscles to recover and enhances training efficiency.
- ○ **Active Rest Days:** Active rest can include low-intensity activities such as light walking, yoga, or stretching. These activities help keep the body moving while supporting recovery.

4. **Example of an Exercise Program Supporting Fat Loss**

The example program below includes a balanced mix of cardio, resistance, and HIIT training on a weekly basis. The program can be adapted to personal needs:

Day	Type of Exercise	Duration/Set	Intensity
Monday	Resistance Training (Full Body)	3 sets x 10 reps	Orta-Yüksek
Tuesday	Cardio (Moderate Intensity)	30-45 minutes	Orta
Wednesday	HIIT	20 minutes	Yüksek
Thursday	Rest or Active Rest	-	-

Friday	Resistance Training (Legs/Lower Body)	3 sets x 10-12 reps	Moderate-High
Saturday	Cardio (Moderate Intensity)	30-45 minutes	Moderate
Sunday	Rest or Light Walking	20-30 minutes	Low

1. **The Combined Effect of Nutrition and Exercise Programs**

   To optimize an exercise program for fat loss, nutrition must also align with the program. Protein intake should be supported to maintain muscle mass, and the ratios of carbohydrates and fats should be balanced. This way, energy levels are maintained while fat loss is supported.

   An exercise program supporting fat loss should include different types of exercises such as cardio, resistance training, and HIIT. The program should progress at a sustainable pace tailored to the individual's physical condition and needs. Attention to rest and recovery processes supports fat loss while preserving overall health.

Methods to Increase Daily Mobility

Today, a sedentary lifestyle has become a common issue, especially for those working desk jobs. Increasing daily mobility is important for supporting fat loss and having positive effects on overall health. In this section, we will discuss simple yet effective methods to enhance mobility that you can easily integrate into your daily life.

1. **Increasing Walking Time During the Day**
   - **Step Count Goal:** Walking at least 10,000 steps per day is a common recommendation to reduce sedentary behavior (Tudor-Locke & Bassett, 2004). You can use a pedometer or a smartwatch to track your daily steps.
   - **Short Walking Breaks:** Avoid sitting for long periods at work or home by taking short walking breaks every hour. This improves circulation and boosts energy levels.
   - **Park Further Away:** By parking your car further away from your workplace or shopping center, you can increase your walking time. This simple habit will naturally increase your daily mobility.
2. **Using Stairs**
   - **Prefer Stairs Over the Elevator:** Using stairs instead of an elevator in daily life increases calorie burning and strengthens muscles. Climbing stairs is an effective cardio and resistance training exercise that works the leg and hip muscles.
   - **Choose Longer Stair Routes:** Once you establish the habit, you can select longer stair routes to increase difficulty. This way, your heart rate increases, and calorie burning accelerates (Boreham et al., 2005).

3. **Office Exercises**
   - **Simple Desk Exercises:** Simple stretching exercises and light weight exercises that target arm muscles can be performed while working at your desk, preventing sedentariness and improving posture. You can lift your legs one at a time to work the quadriceps and strengthen your arm muscles with light resistance bands.
   - **Standing Workstations:** Using a standing workstation allows you to burn more calories throughout the day and reduces your sitting time. Standing while working supports back health and improves overall posture.
4. **Adding Movement to Daily Routines**
   - **Housework and Gardening:** Daily activities such as cleaning and gardening naturally burn calories and increase your mobility. Activities like sweeping, mopping, and rearranging heavy furniture support cardiovascular health and engage the muscles.
   - **Walking While Talking on the Phone:** Walking during phone calls is an easy way to avoid sitting for long periods. By making it a habit to walk during phone conversations, you can increase your daily movement.
5. **Active Transportation Methods**
   - **Walking or Biking:** Walking or biking to work or school is not only an environmentally friendly choice but also an effective way to increase daily mobility. Choosing to walk or bike instead of using public transportation or a car for short distances supports daily calorie expenditure.
   - **Get Off One Stop Early on Public Transport:** If you use public transportation, consider getting off one stop before your destination to take extra steps. This simple method can increase your daily mobility.
6. **The Importance of Progressing with Goals**

   One of the best ways to increase daily mobility is to progress with small goals. For instance, setting short-term goals like increasing exercise duration or step count on certain days of the week can help combat sedentariness and develop a long-term healthy habit. Setting small goals also helps maintain motivation (Marcus et al., 2000).

   There are countless simple ways to increase daily mobility. Small habits and movements integrated into daily routines not only help maintain physical health but also support mental health. An active lifestyle accelerates fat loss while positively impacting metabolic health.

8. Superfoods That Aid in Fat Burning

Natural Foods and Supplements That Support Fat Burning

Natural foods and certain supplements can be quite effective in boosting fat burning and supporting metabolism. However, it is important to combine these products with a balanced diet and regular exercise, without expecting miraculous effects. In this section, we will discuss the effects of natural foods and supplements known to support fat burning.

1. Green Tea and Catechins

- **Thermogenic Effect of Green Tea:** Green tea, with its catechins, especially epigallocatechin gallate (EGCG), can boost metabolism. Catechins promote thermogenesis, increasing energy expenditure and enhancing fat oxidation (Hursel et al., 2009). Studies have shown that regular green tea consumption increases fat burning.
- **Combination of Caffeine and EGCG:** Green tea is also a natural source of caffeine, which helps burn more calories by raising energy levels and supporting the fat-burning process.
- **Catechins and EGCG:** The catechins in green tea, particularly EGCG, exhibit a thermogenic effect, accelerating metabolism and promoting fat oxidation. Research indicates that regular green tea consumption can help reduce body fat (Hursel et al., 2009). EGCG facilitates the breakdown of fat cells, especially aiding in the conversion of abdominal fat into energy.
- **Caffeine Content:** The caffeine in green tea boosts energy levels, helping to burn more calories during physical activity. The combination of caffeine and EGCG in green tea naturally supports the fat-burning process.

2. Ginger

- **Supports Digestive Health:** Ginger is a natural food that aids digestion and supports gut health. The gingerols and shogaols in ginger can create a thermogenic effect, speeding up fat burning (Lahiri et al., 2015).
- **Anti-Inflammatory Effect:** Ginger helps reduce inflammation, enabling the metabolism to work more efficiently, which aids the conversion of body fat into energy.

3. Coffee and Caffeine

- **Release of Fatty Acids:** Coffee, as a natural source of caffeine, helps release fatty acids, accelerating fat burning in the body. Caffeine can temporarily increase metabolism, helping burn more calories (Acheson et al., 1980).
- **Enhances Exercise Performance:** Caffeine taken before exercise can enhance performance, enabling more intense workouts, indirectly supporting fat burning.
- **Metabolic Effect of Caffeine:** Coffee, rich in caffeine, aids in the release of fatty acids and speeds up metabolism. Research shows that caffeine can temporarily increase metabolic rate, allowing for more calorie burning during exercise, supporting fat loss (Acheson et al., 1980).

- **Boosts Performance:** Caffeine enhances exercise performance, enabling more intense workouts, indirectly accelerating fat burning.

4. Hot Peppers and Capsaicin

- **Capsaicin and Thermogenic Effect:** Capsaicin in hot peppers creates a thermogenic effect, supporting calorie burning. Research suggests that capsaicin accelerates metabolism and suppresses appetite (Whiting et al., 2012). Thus, consuming hot peppers in meals contributes to both faster metabolism and satiety.

5. Apple Cider Vinegar

- **Regulates Insulin Levels:** Apple cider vinegar can help control appetite by regulating blood sugar levels. The acetic acid in apple cider vinegar helps reduce fat storage and promotes fat burning (Kondo et al., 2009).
- **Provides Satiety:** Consuming apple cider vinegar before meals delays stomach emptying, leading to longer-lasting fullness, helping reduce calorie intake and supporting fat loss.

6. Protein Supplements

- **Preserves Muscle Mass:** Adequate protein intake is crucial for preserving muscle mass, which keeps metabolism elevated during fat burning. For those engaged in intense training, protein supplements like protein powder support muscle repair, maintaining a higher metabolism.
- **Thermic Effect:** Protein digestion requires more energy than carbohydrates or fats. Therefore, a high-protein diet leads to more calories being burned (Paddon-Jones et al., 2008).

7. Omega-3 Fatty Acids

- **Promotes Fat Burning:** Omega-3 fatty acids from sources like fish oil, chia seeds, and flaxseeds improve metabolism and support fat burning (Buckley & Howe, 2009).
- **Reduces Inflammation:** Omega-3 fatty acids reduce inflammation, aiding in more efficient metabolism. They also speed up muscle recovery after exercise, allowing for quicker return to workouts.

8. High-Fiber Foods

- **Provides Satiety:** Fiber-rich foods (vegetables, fruits, whole grains) delay stomach emptying, leading to prolonged fullness. This is highly effective for controlling calorie intake.

- **Supports Digestive Health:** Fiber supports the digestive system, maintaining gut health. A healthy digestive system contributes to the regulation of fat and energy metabolism.

9. Probiotic Supplements

- **Improves Gut Health:** Probiotics balance gut flora, enhancing digestive health and supporting metabolism. Studies show that probiotics can be effective in reducing belly fat (Kadooka et al., 2010).
- **Appetite Control:** A healthy gut flora helps regulate appetite hormones, supporting weight management.

10. L-Carnitine

- **Converts Fatty Acids into Energy:** L-Carnitine is an amino acid that helps convert fatty acids into energy in cells, accelerating fat burning and boosting energy levels.
- **Supports Exercise Performance:** L-Carnitine supplementation can increase workout endurance, aiding fat burning. However, effects may vary by individual.

Natural foods and certain supplements can support fat burning. However, to fully benefit from these products, a balanced diet and regular exercise habits should be developed. Additionally, consulting a healthcare professional before using any supplements is essential.

Proper Use of Superfoods and Potential Side Effects

"Superfoods" are foods with high nutritional value known for their health benefits. When added to a diet, they can support overall health and help the body achieve goals like fat burning. However, the misuse of some superfoods can lead to side effects or may be incompatible with other health conditions. In this section, we will discuss the benefits, proper usage, and potential side effects of some commonly used superfoods.

1. **Spirulina**

   Benefits: Spirulina is rich in protein, B vitamins, iron, magnesium, and antioxidants. It can accelerate fat burning, boost energy levels, and contains chlorophyll, which aids in detoxification and supports the immune system.

   Proper Use: The recommended daily dose is between 1-3 grams. It can be taken in powder or tablet form, often mixed into smoothies or water. Starting with a low dose helps the body adjust.

   Potential Side Effects: Excessive consumption may cause nausea, headaches, and digestive issues. Spirulina from contaminated sources may carry health risks due to heavy metal exposure. Those with autoimmune diseases should avoid spirulina as it may stimulate the immune system (Raupach et al., 2012).

2. **Chia Seeds**

   Benefits: Chia seeds are high in fiber, omega-3 fatty acids, protein, and antioxidants, which support digestive health and help with satiety, often recommended for weight management and fat loss.

   Proper Use: Chia seeds can be mixed with liquid to form a gel, then added to salads, smoothies, or yogurt. The daily recommended amount is usually 1-2 tablespoons.

   Potential Side Effects: Excessive chia seed intake may lead to gas and bloating due to the high fiber content. As they swell with water, consuming them dry may pose a choking risk, so it's important to soak them first (Jovanovski et al., 2020).

3. **Quinoa**

   Benefits: Quinoa is a complete protein, supporting muscle health and aiding fat loss. It's also rich in iron, magnesium, phosphorus, and fiber, contributing to satiety and weight control.

   Proper Use: Quinoa can be cooked and added to salads, soups, or meals. About one serving, or half a cup of cooked quinoa daily, is considered a balanced amount.

   Potential Side Effects: Quinoa may cause stomach sensitivity or allergic reactions in some individuals. It contains saponins, which have a bitter taste and can be toxic; thoroughly rinsing quinoa before cooking reduces saponin content (Navruz-Varli & Sanlier, 2016).

4. **Turmeric**

   Benefits: Turmeric contains curcumin, known for its anti-inflammatory and antioxidant properties. It can support weight management by inhibiting fat cell development and strengthening the digestive system while aiding detoxification.

   Proper Use: Turmeric can be added to foods, consumed as tea, or taken as a supplement. A daily dose of 1-3 grams is adequate, and pairing with black pepper enhances curcumin absorption.

   Potential Side Effects: Excessive turmeric can cause heartburn, nausea, and dizziness. Individuals with gallbladder issues should avoid turmeric, as it may increase bile production (Cheng et al., 2020).

5. **Matcha Tea**

   Benefits: Matcha tea is rich in catechins and antioxidants, which boost metabolism and support fat burning. Additionally, the L-theanine content in matcha has stress-reducing effects.

Proper Use: Consuming 1-2 teaspoons of matcha powder mixed with water or added to smoothies daily is recommended, ideally in the morning or before a high-energy activity.

Potential Side Effects: Excess matcha consumption may increase caffeine intake, leading to sleep issues, anxiety, and digestive discomfort. In some individuals, the high antioxidant concentration may cause dizziness or nausea when consumed in large amounts (Kim et al., 2017).

Superfoods and certain supplements can support fat burning, but to fully benefit from their effects, a balanced diet and regular exercise are essential. It's also important to consult a healthcare professional before using any supplement.

9. Lifestyle Tips for Sustainable Nutrition and Fat Burning

Developing Healthy Habits and Maintaining a Nutritional Routine

Maintaining a healthy lifestyle requires strong commitment, both mentally and physically, for long-term success. Achieving sustainable change in eating habits is possible by adopting healthy habits that can be practiced for life, rather than relying on quick fixes. In this section, we will explore the scientific basis of forming healthy habits, methods for sustaining motivation, and strategies for maintaining your nutritional routine.

1. **The Science of Building Healthy Habits** Habit formation is the process of turning a conscious behavior into an automatic one through repetition. It typically takes about 66 days for habits to become established, so patience is essential when creating new habits (Lally et al., 2010). Key strategies to support habit formation include:
   - **Taking Small Steps:** Begin with small, manageable goals instead of large changes. For instance, adding healthy options to one meal a day or increasing water intake can lay the foundation for significant changes.
   - **Cue and Reward Cycle:** Every habit relies on a trigger (e.g., waking up), a routine (e.g., drinking water), and a reward (e.g., feeling more energized). Identify triggers that help you stick to your habits.
   - **Automating Routines:** Creating a regular meal plan or weekly exercise schedule helps integrate healthy choices into your life more easily. Over time, these routines become simpler to follow.

2. **Maintaining and Regaining Motivation** Motivation is key to sustaining a healthy eating routine, though it can fluctuate. To make motivation more sustainable, use the following strategies to support your goals and progress:
   - **Set Short- and Long-Term Goals:** Break long-term goals into short-term, achievable ones. For example, instead of aiming to "lose 10 kg in 6 months," start with a short-term goal like "prepare healthy meals three times this week" for more sustainable progress.
   - **Track Your Progress:** Make your progress visible by celebrating small wins. Keeping a journal or recording achievements can enhance motivation.
   - **Build Support Systems:** Family members, friends, or support groups with similar goals can be valuable sources of motivation. Such systems strengthen your journey toward a healthy lifestyle and provide morale.

3. **Strategies for Sustaining a Nutritional Routine** To sustain healthy eating habits in the long term, the following strategies can be helpful:
   - **Mindful and Planned Food Choices:** Creating a weekly meal plan can help you make healthy choices for each meal. Preparing healthy snacks in advance also helps prevent poor choices during hunger.
   - **Sticking to Meal Routines:** Skipping meals, especially breakfast, can lead to cravings throughout the day. Regular meals help balance blood sugar and prevent sudden hunger.
   - **Prioritizing Food Variety:** To obtain the vitamins, minerals, and macronutrients your body needs, include a variety of foods in your diet. Different-colored fruits and vegetables, protein sources, and whole grains are essential for balanced nutrition.
   - **Allowing Flexibility:** Instead of feeling restricted or guilty, allow occasional indulgences in your diet. Flexibility makes a healthy lifestyle more sustainable.
   - **Paying Attention to Mental Health:** Mental factors like stress management and sleep routine also impact your nutrition. In stressful moments, there may be a tendency to turn to unhealthy foods, so learning stress management techniques is important.

4. **Self-Awareness and Personalizing Habits** Everyone's metabolism, energy needs, and lifestyle vary. Recognizing your unique needs is essential in the process of healthy eating and habit formation. Listening to your body's signals and personalizing habits according to your needs can help sustain them in the long term.

Developing healthy habits and maintaining a nutritional routine is a lifelong journey rather than a short-term effort. Starting with small steps, being patient and flexible with yourself, and setting goals that suit you will make healthy habits more permanent. Creating motivation sources and supporting your healthy food choices are keys to enhancing your quality of life.

Nutrition in Social Life: Making Healthy Choices While Dining Out
Maintaining a healthy diet requires making mindful choices not only at home but also when eating out and participating in social gatherings. Dining in restaurants or attending social events can be challenging for those committed to a balanced diet. However, with conscious decisions, it's possible to stick to a healthy eating plan even in social settings. This section explores tips for making healthy choices while dining out, managing nutrition in social situations, and aligning a healthy eating plan with social life.

1. Key Principles for Making Healthy Choices While Dining Out

Use these strategies to make healthier choices when eating out:

- **Review the Menu in Advance**: Check the restaurant's menu beforehand to identify healthy options. Many restaurants now offer online menus with healthier choices, which can help you make quicker decisions and avoid high-calorie dishes.
- **Control Portion Sizes**: Restaurant portions are often large. Share a meal, order a half portion, or take leftovers home to control portion sizes. This helps avoid unnecessary calorie intake.
- **Pay Attention to Preparation Methods**: The way food is prepared affects its calorie and nutrient content. Choose options that are grilled, baked, steamed, or boiled instead of fried. For salads, consider ordering dressings on the side to control calorie intake.
- **Opt for Protein and Fiber Sources**: To stay full longer, choose options that include protein (chicken, fish, meat) and fiber-rich foods (vegetables, whole grains). These help stabilize blood sugar and prevent sudden hunger.

2. Healthy Eating Strategies for Social Situations

Apply these simple yet effective strategies to eat healthily in social settings:

- **Avoid Going Hungry**: Have a light snack or a protein-rich small meal before an event to avoid arriving hungry. This can prevent overeating.
- **Suggest Healthy Alternatives**: When ordering food at a gathering or choosing a restaurant, suggest healthier options. This makes it easier for both you and others to make healthy choices.
- **Avoid Sugary Beverages**: Opt for water, mineral water, or unsweetened drinks instead of sugary or alcoholic beverages, which keep calorie intake low while supporting hydration.
- **Eat Slowly and Listen to Fullness Cues**: Eating slowly while conversing helps you recognize fullness signals, reducing the risk of overeating before you feel overly full.

3. Balancing Social Life and Healthy Eating

Maintaining a healthy lifestyle doesn't require withdrawing from social life. On the contrary, engaging in activities that support social connections can uplift morale and motivation. To balance the two:

- **Plan Ahead**: For special events or holidays, make healthier choices instead of abandoning healthy habits entirely. For example, load up your plate with vegetables and protein at a buffet or have just a taste of dessert.
- **Avoid Excessive Restrictions**: Healthy eating is about balance; constant restriction can lead to stress in social situations. Allowing for occasional indulgences makes it easier to stick to a healthy eating pattern in the long term.
- **Incorporate Healthy Living into Social Activities**: Bring your healthy choices into your social circle. Suggest a healthy restaurant or a walk with friends, which adds a healthy touch to social activities while making your lifestyle more sustainable.

4. Developing Decision-Making Skills in Social Settings

Strengthening willpower and making mindful choices in social environments are key to maintaining healthy habits. Developing these skills can help you feel more confident in making healthy choices:

- **Remember Your Goals**: When presented with unhealthy options, remember how making healthy choices contributes to your long-term goals. This awareness can support better decisions.
- **Celebrate Your Successes**: Recognize and appreciate when you make healthy choices in social settings. Positive reinforcement helps make these habits more sustainable.

Maintaining healthy eating habits in social life is possible, and these habits not only improve your quality of life but also support a lifestyle that aligns well with your social relationships. Making conscious choices allows for a more flexible and enjoyable experience in social environments while helping you sustain a healthy lifestyle.

Long-Term Motivation and Goal-Setting Methods

Staying motivated in long-term goals like weight loss, fat burning, or adopting a healthy lifestyle is often one of the biggest challenges. While motivation may be strong at the beginning, it can fade over time, making it essential to implement effective strategies to maintain commitment. In this section, we'll explore ways to set long-term goals and sustain motivation, sharing tips that will keep you on track toward success.

1. **Setting Realistic and Achievable Goals** The first step to success is setting realistic and attainable goals. Ensuring that your goals are challenging but achievable helps you sustain motivation over time.
   - **Use SMART Goals**: The SMART (Specific, Measurable, Achievable, Relevant, Time-Bound) method helps you stay focused when setting your goals. For instance, setting a measurable and time-bound goal like "losing 5 kg in six months" offers a clear path forward.
   - **Progress with Small Steps**: Breaking down a distant goal into smaller, more attainable milestones makes it easier to track your progress. Setting weekly or monthly targets, like small weight loss increments, leads to a big change over time.

2. **Connecting Goals to Your 'Why'** When setting goals, consider why you want to achieve them. A strong reason forms the foundation of motivation and keeps you committed during challenging times.
   - **Find a Strong 'Why'**: Go beyond superficial goals like losing weight and think about personal and meaningful reasons, like improving energy levels or boosting self-confidence.
   - **Write It Down**: Recording your reasons in a journal or digital notepad allows you to revisit them when motivation wanes. Reflecting on these reasons can renew your resolve when needed.

3. **Tracking Progress and Rewarding Yourself** Seeing your progress can be incredibly motivating. By tracking your journey and celebrating small successes, you can keep your motivation fresh.
   - **Regular Monitoring**: Track your progress by recording body measurements, tracking weight changes, comparing photos, or measuring workout performance. These records provide tangible evidence of your progress, helping sustain motivation over time.
   - **Reward Yourself with Small Treats**: Reward yourself whenever you reach a small milestone. These rewards reinforce your commitment to your goals. For instance, treating yourself to a shopping trip or new sportswear can keep your motivation alive.

4. **Building Routines and Developing Discipline** Even when motivation fades over time, a disciplined routine will lead you to your goals. Integrating healthy habits into daily life makes them more sustainable.

   - **Incorporate Healthy Habits into Your Daily Routine**: Adding habits like morning walks, regular exercise, drinking enough water, or scheduled meal times positively impacts your lifestyle.
   - **Prioritize Discipline**: Successful people don't just rely on motivation; they work with discipline. Discipline is essential for establishing habits and creating a consistent lifestyle.

5. **Getting Support and Shaping Your Environment** Social support plays a significant role in achieving long-term goals. Getting support from people around you can help you maintain motivation.

   - **Create a Supportive Environment**: Surrounding yourself with friends or family members who are also focused on healthy living can boost your motivation. Staying connected with people who support your goals makes it easier to overcome challenges.
   - **Seek Professional Help**: Working with a dietitian, trainer, or life coach allows you to plan your goals more professionally. These individuals guide you toward your objectives and help maintain motivation.

6. **Accepting the Process of Change and Progress** Achieving goals can sometimes take longer than expected. During these times, focusing on the process and being patient with yourself is crucial.

   - **Remember That Change is a Process**: Lifestyle changes require patience and continuity. Accepting that short-term setbacks don't hinder long-term success helps you stay positive and trust the process.
   - **Don't Underestimate the Power of Small Changes**: Remember that daily small changes can lead to significant results over time. This approach not only helps maintain motivation but also makes healthy habits more sustainable.

7. **Knowing Yourself and Reframing Challenges** Self-awareness is essential on a long-term goal journey. Learning about your strengths, weaknesses, and how to handle challenges helps you stay motivated.

- o **Identify What Motivates You**: Discover what motivates you and keep reminding yourself of it. For example, keeping a success journal and noting your progress allows you to revisit these sources of motivation frequently.
- o **See Obstacles as Opportunities**: Every challenge is a chance to learn and grow. View setbacks as temporary and move forward by learning from them, emerging stronger each time.

Long-term motivation and goal-setting methods provide a guide to support your journey to success. Accepting that reaching your goals can take time boosts your self-confidence and leads to more sustainable success. Integrating healthy habits into your life allows you to achieve significant results through small steps.

Adapting to a Nutrition and Exercise Routine

Adopting a healthy lifestyle often requires balancing both nutrition and exercise habits. However, integrating these habits into daily life can sometimes be challenging. In this section, we'll explore ways to adapt to a nutrition and exercise routine and examine the essential steps for a successful lifestyle.

1. Setting Goals

The first step in establishing a sustainable nutrition and exercise routine is to set clear, achievable goals.

- **Set Specific Goals:** Define your goals clearly. For instance, setting concrete goals like "exercise three times a week" or "drink 2 liters of water every day" makes tracking progress easier.
- **Short- and Long-Term Goals:** Establishing both short-term goals (e.g., losing 2 kilograms in one month) and long-term goals (e.g., losing 10 kilograms in six months) keeps motivation high and helps monitor progress.

2. Planning and Preparation

Good planning is a key factor in successful adaptation to routines.

- **Create a Weekly Plan:** Ease the preparation process by planning your exercises and meals for each week. Knowing what you'll do on which days helps maintain discipline.
- **Make a Shopping List:** Prepare a shopping list filled with healthy ingredients to reduce the chances of buying unhealthy foods. Shopping according to this list can help establish a regular nutrition routine.

3. Start with Small Changes

Taking small, sustainable steps instead of making big changes all at once can make adaptation easier.

- **Break Down Habits:** Instead of trying to change everything at once, add a new habit each week. For example, in the first week, add a daily fruit, and in the second week, try exercising twice a week.
- **Start with Small Portions:** When adjusting eating habits, starting with smaller portions helps your body adjust and supports the formation of habits.

4. Maintaining High Motivation

Sustaining motivation makes it easier to make healthy lifestyle changes permanent.

- **Track Your Progress:** Seeing the progress you've made boosts motivation. Track weight changes, exercise times, or healthy food intake by keeping a journal or using an app.
- **Join Support Groups:** Meeting with people who have similar goals can boost your motivation. Exercise classes or nutrition groups offer both support and a sense of accountability.

5. Making Your Routine Flexible

Life can sometimes be unpredictable, and flexibility plays a crucial role in adapting.

- **Review Your Plans:** While trying to stick to your plans, don't forget to show flexibility when necessary. If you miss a day of exercise, make an extra effort on other days to compensate.
- **Adapt to Changing Conditions:** If changes occur due to work, social life, or other responsibilities, create a new plan. Simple adjustments, like shifting workouts to mornings or evenings, can help you stay on track.

6. Making it Enjoyable and Fun

Turning your nutrition and exercise routine into something enjoyable increases adherence.

- **Make Exercise Fun:** Try different activities to make your exercises more enjoyable. Activities like dancing, group sports, or hiking can energize your routine.
- **Enjoy the Meal Prep Process:** Make meal preparation fun by trying new healthy recipes or cooking with friends, making healthy eating habits more enjoyable.

7. Rewarding Yourself

Celebrating your achievements increases motivation and strengthens your commitment to your goals.

- **Set Small Rewards:** When you reach your goals, reward yourself with small treats. New workout gear, a fun day out, or a favorite activity can help keep you motivated.
- **Celebrate Successes:** Celebrate achievements like weight loss or completing a new exercise program to encourage yourself. These celebrations not only keep you focused on your goals but also boost your motivation.

Adapting to a nutrition and exercise routine requires discipline and determination. Setting goals, planning, starting with small changes, and maintaining high motivation are essential steps in this journey. Embracing flexibility and a fun approach can make it easier to sustain a healthy lifestyle. Enjoy your achievements and make your healthy habits permanent!

Sample Meal Plans and Shopping Lists

To adopt a healthy lifestyle, it's essential to create a balanced meal plan and gather the necessary ingredients. Below are sample weekly meal plans and corresponding shopping lists.

Sample Meal Plan

Day 1

- Breakfast: Oatmeal with milk, fresh fruit, and walnuts
- Snack: Yogurt and a handful of almonds
- Lunch: Grilled chicken breast with quinoa salad (tomato, cucumber, parsley)
- Snack: Carrots and hummus
- Dinner: Baked salmon with broccoli and sweet potatoes

Day 2

- Breakfast: Smoothie (spinach, banana, almond milk, chia seeds)
- Snack: Whole wheat bread with avocado
- Lunch: Lentil soup with whole wheat bread
- Snack: Fresh fruit (apple or pear)
- Dinner: Chicken fajita (tortilla, bell pepper, onion) with green salad

Day 3

- Breakfast: 2 boiled eggs, whole wheat bread, tomatoes, and olives
- Snack: Milk and a handful of walnuts
- Lunch: Quinoa salad (chickpeas, corn, lemon dressing)
- Snack: Yogurt with a tablespoon of honey
- Dinner: Grilled vegetable stuffed eggplant (eggplant, zucchini) with bulgur pilaf

Shopping List

Protein Sources

- Chicken breast (500 g)
- Salmon (300 g)
- Eggs (12)
- Yogurt (500 g)
- Chickpeas (canned or dried)
- Lentils (dried)

Grains and Legumes

- Oatmeal (500 g)
- Quinoa (250 g)
- Whole wheat bread (1 loaf)
- Bulgur (250 g)
- Chia seeds (100 g)

Vegetables

- Tomatoes (4)
- Cucumbers (2)
- Carrots (4)
- Broccoli (1 head)
- Bell peppers (3 - red, green, yellow)
- Spinach (1 bunch)
- Eggplants (2)
- Zucchini (2)
- Sweet potatoes (2)

Fruits

- Bananas (4)
- Apples (4)
- Pears (4)
- Fresh seasonal fruit

Nuts and Seeds

- Walnuts (200 g)
- Almonds (200 g)

Oils

- Olive oil (500 ml)
- Avocados (2)

Spices and Condiments

- Salt
- Black pepper
- Red pepper
- Lemon juice

Additional Tips

- **Meal Prep:** Preparing meals at the beginning of the week makes healthy eating easier. For example, you can cook vegetables and proteins in bulk for several meals in one day.
- **Portion Control:** When shopping, pay attention to portion sizes. Overbuying can negatively impact healthy eating habits.
- **Fresh Ingredients:** Choose seasonal and fresh fruits and vegetables; they're rich in nutrients and taste great.

This meal plan and shopping list will help you build balanced eating habits. Always remember to adjust it to fit your needs and taste preferences!

Healthy Recipes and Tips

Eating healthy is important for both maintaining body health and supporting fat loss. Below are some healthy recipes and related tips.

Oatmeal Breakfast
Ingredients:

- 1 cup oatmeal
- 2 cups milk (or almond milk)
- 1 banana
- 1 tablespoon chia seeds
- 1 teaspoon cinnamon
- A handful of walnuts or almonds

Instructions:

- o   Place the oatmeal and milk in a saucepan and cook over medium heat.
- o   When it starts to boil, add cinnamon and chia seeds.
- o   Stir the mixture until it thickens.
- o   Serve with sliced banana and walnuts or almonds on top.

Tip: You can prepare this breakfast the night before and store it in the refrigerator. You can also enhance the flavor by adding different fruits or yogurt.

Grilled Chicken Salad
Ingredients:

- o   200 g chicken breast
- o   1 cup leafy greens (arugula, lettuce, spinach)
- o   1/2 cup cherry tomatoes
- o   1/2 cucumber
- o   1/4 cup feta cheese
- o   2 tablespoons olive oil
- o   Lemon juice
- o   Salt and pepper

Instructions:

- o   Marinate the chicken breast with olive oil, salt, and pepper, then cook it on a grill or pan.
- o   For the salad, combine leafy greens, cherry tomatoes, and chopped cucumber in a bowl.
- o   Slice the cooked chicken and add it to the salad.
- o   Sprinkle feta cheese on top and drizzle with lemon juice.

Tip: You can try different protein sources like turkey, tuna, or chickpeas instead of chicken.

Baked Salmon and Vegetables
Ingredients:

- o   300 g salmon fillet
- o   1 zucchini
- o   1 carrot
- o   1/2 head of broccoli
- o   2 tablespoons olive oil
- o   1 teaspoon lemon zest

- ○ Salt, pepper, and fresh herbs (thyme, dill)

Instructions:

- ○ Preheat the oven to 180°C (350°F).
- ○ Place the salmon fillet on a baking sheet and arrange the vegetables (zucchini, carrot, broccoli) around it.
- ○ Add olive oil, lemon zest, salt, pepper, and fresh herbs on top.
- ○ Bake for 20-25 minutes.

Tip: You can substitute salmon with other types of fish or chicken. Feel free to vary the vegetables to your preference.

Chia Seed Pudding
Ingredients:

- ○ 1/4 cup chia seeds
- ○ 1 cup milk (or plant-based milk)
- ○ 1 tablespoon honey or maple syrup
- ○ 1/2 teaspoon vanilla extract
- ○ Fresh fruit (e.g., strawberries or blueberries)

Instructions:

- ○ In a bowl, mix chia seeds, milk, honey, and vanilla extract.
- ○ Let the mixture sit in the refrigerator for at least 2 hours or overnight.
- ○ Serve with fresh fruit on top.

Tip: You can add variety by using different fruits, nuts, or types of seeds.

Smart Snacks

- ○ **Yogurt and Fresh Fruit:** A mix of low-fat yogurt and fresh fruit satisfies your sweet cravings and supports protein intake.
- ○ **Carrot Sticks and Hummus:** Carrot sticks make a perfect snack when paired with hummus. Nutritious and filling!
- ○ **Nut Mix:** A mix of almonds, walnuts, and hazelnuts provides healthy fats and protein. Just be mindful of portion sizes.

Healthy recipes and tips are essential parts of a balanced diet plan. By enriching your daily meals with these recipes, you can adopt a lifestyle that's both healthy and delicious. Don't forget to personalize the recipes to match your taste!

Conclusion: The Results of Your Healthy Living Journey

"The Nutrition and Fat Burning Guide" aims to be your companion on your journey to healthy living. The information presented in this book is designed to help you gain a deep understanding of healthy eating, exercise, and lifestyle changes. The most important thing to remember is that this journey is a marathon, and every individual progresses at their own pace.

The potential for improving your quality of life through developing and maintaining healthy habits is immense. When setting your goals, taking the necessary steps to achieve those goals is the first step towards adopting a healthy lifestyle. Remember, making small changes each day can lead to significant results over time.

There is a strong connection between mental and physical health. Be kind to yourself, enjoy the process, and view your setbacks as opportunities to learn. It is essential to regularly practice stress management techniques, establish a good sleep routine, and take time for yourself to maintain your mental health.

In this journey, seeking support and sharing with others can enhance your motivation. Family members, friends, or communities can be by your side to support your healthy living goals. Working together not only increases your sense of accountability but also helps you enjoy your journey.

Remember that healthy living is not just a physical goal but a lifestyle. We hope that with what you've learned in this book, you possess the knowledge and motivation necessary to maintain a healthy life. By aiming to take one more step towards health every day, you can begin to lead a healthier and happier life.

We wish you success on your healthy living journey! May you experience every moment of your life in a healthy and meaningful way.

References

American College of Sports Medicine. (2021). *ACSM's Guidelines for Exercise Testing and Prescription*. 10th ed. Philadelphia: Wolters Kluwer.

Centers for Disease Control and Prevention. (2020). *Overweight and Obesity*. [Online] Available at:
https://www.cdc.gov/obesity/index.html [Accessed: 5 Nov 2024].

Harvard T.H. Chan School of Public Health. (n.d.). *Healthy Eating Plate*. [Online] Available at: https://www.hsph.harvard.edu/nutritionsource/healthy-eating-plate/ [Accessed: 5 Nov 2024].

Kahn, S.E., Hull, R.L., and Utzschneider, K.M. (2006). "Insulin Resistance and Its Role in the Pathogenesis of Type 2 Diabetes Mellitus." *Journal of Clinical Endocrinology & Metabolism*, 91(7): 2467-2470.

National Institutes of Health. (2013). *Clinical Guidelines on the Identification, Evaluation, and Treatment of Overweight and Obesity in Adults: The Evidence Report*. Obesity Research, 6(Suppl 2): 51S-209S.

Phillips, S.M., and Van Loon, L.J.C. (2011). "Dietary Protein for Athletes: From Requirements to Metabolism." *Journal of Sports Sciences*, 29(1): 3-13.

Puhl, R.M., and Heuer, C.A. (2010). "Obesity Stigma: A Review of the Evidence and Implications for Public Health." *Health Education & Behavior*, 37(5): 634-647.

USDA. (2020). *Dietary Guidelines for Americans 2020-2025*. 9th ed. Washington, DC: U.S. Department of Agriculture.

Volpi, E., Kobayashi, H., and Sheffield-Moore, M. (2001). "Essential Amino Acids and Muscle Protein Recovery from Resistance Exercise." *The American Journal of Clinical Nutrition*, 74(4): 540-548.

World Health Organization. (2021). *Healthy Diet*. [Online] Available at: https://www.who.int/news-room/fact-sheets/detail/healthy-diet [Accessed: 5 Nov 2024].

Zorba, E. (2018). "The Role of Omega-3 Fatty Acids in Weight Loss: A Review." *Nutrition Reviews*, 76(10): 749-761.